Port Surgery

Springer Nature More Media App

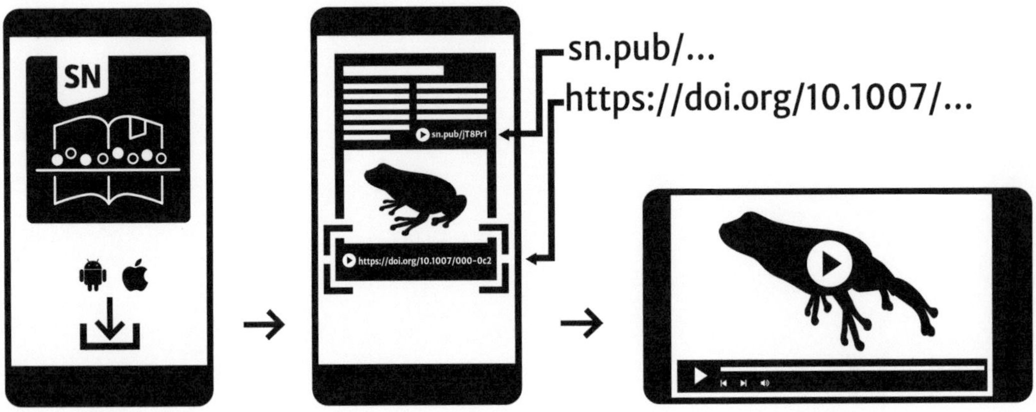

1. Download **2. Scan Link** **3. Enjoy Video**

Support: customerservice@springernature.com

Roland Hennes
Editor

Port Surgery

Implantation and Explantation Procedures in Practice and Clinic

Springer

Editor
Roland Hennes
Klinik für Allgemein-, Viszeral- und Transplantationschirurgie
Universitätsklinikum Heidelberg
Heidelberg, Germany

This work contains media enhancements, which are displayed with a "play" icon. Material in the print book can be viewed on a mobile device by downloading the "Springer Nature More Media" app available in the major app stores. The media enhancements in the online version of the work can be accessed directly by authorized users.

ISBN 978-3-662-70623-7 ISBN 978-3-662-70624-4 (eBook)
https://doi.org/10.1007/978-3-662-70624-4

Translation from the German language edition: "Port-Operationen" by Roland Hennes, © Der/die Herausgeber bzw. der/die Autor(en), exklusiv lizenziert an Springer-Verlag GmbH, DE, ein Teil von Springer Nature 2024. Published by Springer Berlin Heidelberg. All Rights Reserved.

This book is a translation of the original German edition "Port-Operationen" by Roland Hennes, published by Springer-Verlag GmbH, DE in 2024. The translation was done with the help of an artificial intelligence machine translation tool. A subsequent human revision was done primarily in terms of content, so that the book will read stylistically differently from a conventional translation. Springer Nature works continuously to further the development of tools for the production of books and on the related technologies to support the authors.

This Springer imprint is published by the registered company Springer-Verlag GmbH, DE, part of Springer Nature.
The registered company address is: Heidelberger Platz 3, 14197 Berlin, Germany

Foreword

For 18 years, Prof. Hennes has been continuously developing surgical techniques for central venous catheters, particularly for ports. This led to the establishment of the Port Center at the Department of Surgery, University Hospital Heidelberg—the first of its kind at a university hospital worldwide. He has successfully managed this Port Center since 2011, drawing on the experience of 20,000 port procedures performed personally. Several studies conducted by the Clinical Trials Center of the Department of Surgery at University Hospital Heidelberg have enabled the applied surgical techniques for ports to be reviewed and evaluated.

His extensive knowledge of central venous catheter surgical techniques and the development of alternative and microsurgical procedures increase the success rate, minimize intra- and postoperative complications, and improve the quality of life for port carriers. His focus is not limited to surgical techniques; he has also dedicated a textbook to port care, co-authored with Ms. Gisela Müller, Head of Nursing at the Department of Surgery, University Hospital Heidelberg.

Both a standardized, evidence-based surgical technique and equally professional care of port patients provide the comprehensive context for a satisfied and competently treated patient.

I wish this textbook the success it deserves, given the importance of this topic for the care of our oncology and nutrition patients.

Prof. Dr. med. Christoph Michalski
Universitätsklinik Heidelberg, Chirurgische Klinik

Preface

Since the initial description of the port catheter by Niederhuber in 1982, ports as central venous catheters have played a central role in the treatment of oncologic patients over the past 40 years. They are of similar importance for all patients requiring long-term parenteral nutrition.

Compared to other central venous catheters, such as Hickman, CVC, and PICC lines, port catheters offer distinct advantages. Ports facilitate the highest level of patient quality oflife as virtually all physical activities and sports, such as swimming, cross-country skiing, and tennis, to name a few, can be performed without restriction. They can remain in the body for at least five years before removal or replacement is necessary due to material fatigue. However, one of the most important aspects for patients is the much lower infection rate compared to all other catheters.

To realize all these benefits, standardized and evidence-based surgical techniques are necessary.

Especially for our patients with complex vascular conditions, secondary interventions or re-interventions, and tumors that, hinder port placement in the thoracic region, alternative surgical methods and techniques are necessary.

The appreciation for these procedures is, surprisingly, often very low in light of these demands, even within surgery and other disciplines performing port operations. They are frequently dismissed as a "minor" intervention, intended to be performed as the "last item" of the surgical day by the most junior assistant.

Whatever perspective one may take, the standards of excellence required in surgery must also be demanded and implemented in central venous catheter surgery. It is hoped that this textbook will serve as both an inspiration and a support in this regard.

The quality of life and survival of patients depend critically on the implementation of excellence in this type of surgery.

This is accompanied by competent care of port patients.

In this context, constructive interdisciplinary collaboration among all professional groups involved is essential for the planning and standardized execution of surgical procedures.

All measures and action-oriented steps serve to ensure competent and professional care for patients who are facing the greatest challenges due to their cancer diagnoses.

It is the privilege of surgeons to make a difference for the needs and satisfaction of these patients, ultimately improving the quality of care.

Roland Hennes

Contents

Editor and Contributors

About the Editor

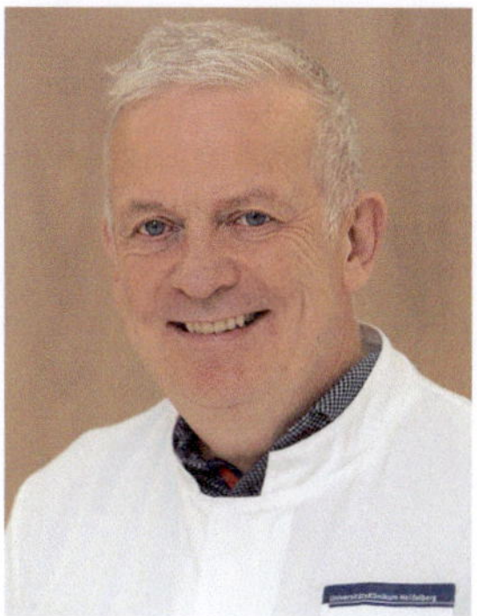

Prof. Dr. med. Roland Hennes Director of the Heidelberg Port Center.

Prof. Dr. med. Roland Hennes founded the world's first port center at a university hospital in 2011. In collaboration with the German Study Center of the Department of Surgery at Heidelberg University Hospital, he was able to further develop surgical techniques based on evidence and establish new microsurgical procedures.

He pursues a holistic approach to the treatment of port patients in order to improve patient care and quality of life. Through the National Tumor Center and other clinics at Heidelberg University Hospital, he has gained extensive experience with many thousands of port patients over 18 years and has developed surgical expertise through more than 20,000 port procedures.

Contributors

Karoline Bleymehl Klinik für Anästhesiologie, Universitätsklinikum Heidelberg, Heidelberg, Deutschland

Prof. Dr. med. De-Hua Chang Radiologie und Nuklearmedizin, Kantonsspital Luzern, Luzern, Schweiz

Dr. med. Vanessa Eichel Sektion für Krankenhaus-und Umwelthygiene, Zentrum für Infektiologie, Universitätsklinikum Heidelberg, Heidelberg, Deutschland

Prof. Dr. Reinhart T. Grundmann Arzt für Chirurgie, Unfallchirurgie, Gefäßchirurgie, Medizinischer Sachverständiger, Burghausen, Deutschland

Dr. med. Dipl.-Ing. Hans Haindl Sachverständiger für Medizintechnik, Wennigsen, Deutschland

Dr. med. Roland Hennes Klinik für Allgemein-, Viszeral- und Transplantationschirurgie, Universitätsklinikum Heidelberg, Heidelberg, Deutschland

Felix Johannes Jost Universitätsklinikum Heidelberg, Heidelberg, Deutschland

Alexander Daniel Wollkopf Institut für Hygiene und Public Health, Universitätsklinikum Bonn, Bonn, Deutschland

Part I

Fundamentals and Preoperative Preparation

1 Basics and Significance of Central Venous Catheters and the Role of Port Catheters

Roland Hennes

> Central venous catheters have always played a prominent role in both inpatient and outpatient care for cancer and nutrition patients. In this chapter, we will briefly discuss the most important central venous catheters, which include the CVC, the Hickman catheter, the Demers catheter, the PICC catheter, and port catheters.

Central venous catheters differ in their structure and function, resulting in various applications. While some indications overlap, the individual needs of each patient must always be considered.

The access routes for central venous catheters include the internal and external jugular veins, the subclavian vein, the cephalic vein in the area of the deltopectoral groove, the basilic vein in the arm, the cephalic vein in the region of the antecubital fossa, the brachial vein, and the femoral vein with its tributaries.

Preferred access routes have been established depending on the type of catheter.

Central venous catheters are now indispensable in clinical care, especially for oncologic patients and those requiring supportive parenteral feeding. Their use however carries risks for the patient if strict hygiene measures are not observed during care and handling, and if staff are not properly trained (Needleman et al. 2002). These risks primarily include systemic and local infections, which can be introduced into the body via the bloodstream or lead to catheter-related infections through septic dissemination (Hennes and Müller 2021; Bundesgesundheitsbl 2017).

1.1 Port Catheters

Port catheters have been known since Niederhuber established ports in clinical practice in the 1990s. Since then, port catheters have been further developed in terms of material and high-pressure capability.

A port catheter consists of a port chamber, a connecting mechanism, and the port catheter itself (Figs. 1.1 and 1.2).

At the Port Center in Heidelberg, only high-pressure ports have been used for the past 12 years. These ports can withstand a flow rate of 5 ml/s, which makes them suitable for contrast agent administration during CT and MRI examinations. This feature is a major advantage, especially for oncology patients who now routinely undergo CT and/or MRI for staging in a modern setting. Port catheters can be used in MRI scanners up to 3 T with the needle in place.

R. Hennes (✉)
Klinik für Allgemein-, Viszeral- und Transplantationschirurgie, Universitätsklinikum Heidelberg, Heidelberg, Germany
e-mail: Roland.Hennes@med.uni-heidelberg.de

R. Hennes (ed.), *Port Surgery*, https://doi.org/10.1007/978-3-662-70624-4_1

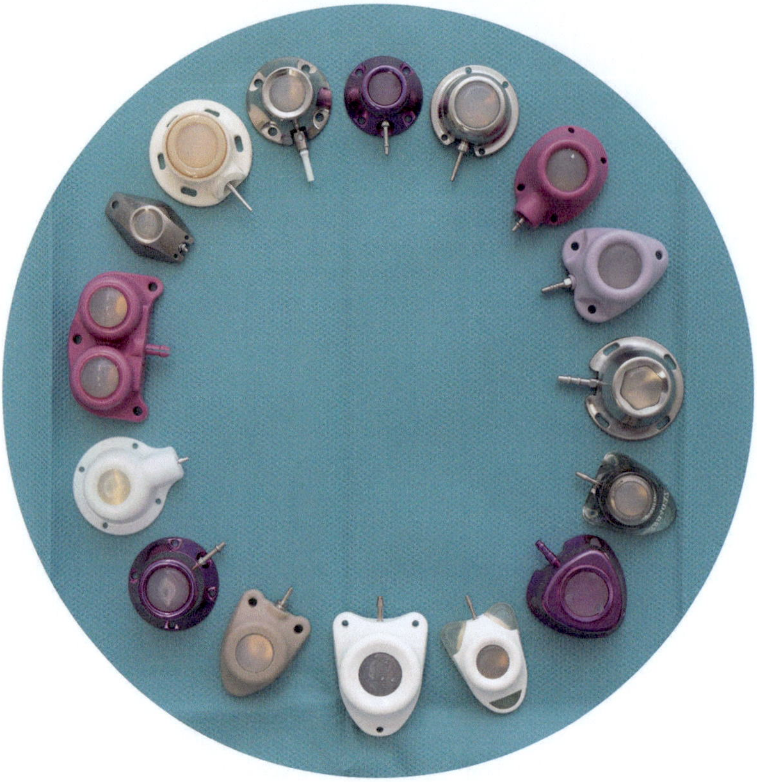

Fig. 1.1 Port chambers in various sizes and designs. (© R. Hennes; all rights reserved)

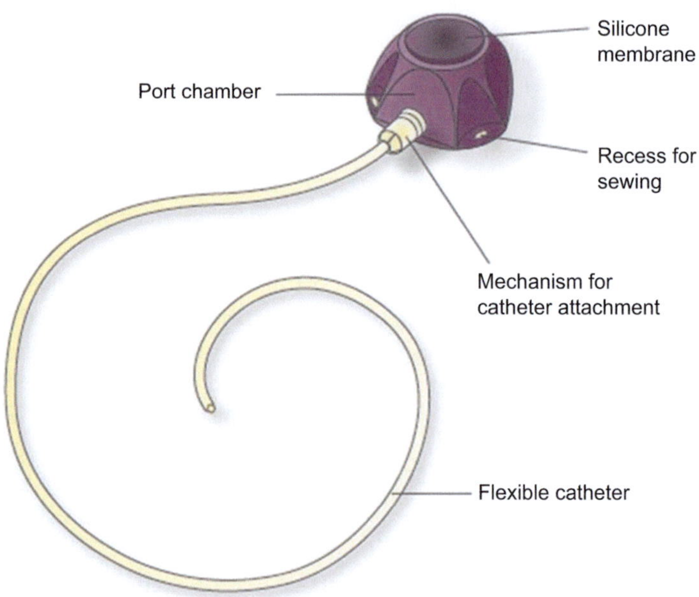

Fig. 1.2 Structure of a port catheter system. (© R. Hennes; all rights reserved)

They can remain in the body for years and thus have the longest dwell time of all central venous catheters.

Even ports that have remained in a patient's body for over 10 years have almost all continued to function well. However, material fatigue is more frequently observed in these cases, manifesting as cracks and other issues. Therefore, removal or replacement of ports is advised after 5 years (see Chap. 3 Materials).

Compared to all other central venous catheters, port catheters offer patients the best quality of life. In fact, all sports and physical activities can be performed without restriction.

Because the implant is located entirely in the subcutaneous tissue, the risk of catheter-related infection originating from a cutaneous entry site is markedly reduced. External infection occurs exclusively via use of the port catheter and puncture of the port chamber. As with all catheters, strict hygiene must be observed during care to prevent infections.

As described above, patients with central venous catheters may also develop infections through septic dissemination via the bloodstream.

1.1.1 Selection of Port Chambers and Port Catheters and Consideration of Cosmetic Aspects

Through thousands of conversations with port patients, especially women with gynecological diseases, the need for a good cosmetic outcome and a port chamber size adapted to the patient's body habitus has become clear.

At the Port Center, we use five different port chamber sizes, which we tailor individually to the depth of the soft tissue mantle.

For port catheters, we use sizes of 6.6 F, 7.5 F, and 9 F.

The 9 F catheter is part of an apheresis port, which is used therapeutically for "blood purification." Almost all therapies can be administered via a 6.6 Fr catheter.

We pay close attention to the size of the incision and the cosmetic result. Of course, it is important for all patients that there is no stigmatization due to the port chamber or the catheter tract being visible through the skin (see the relevant chapters on implantation via venous section). The incision technique and material selection are described in more detail there.

1.1.2 Summary: Port Catheters

Based on the experience at Heidelberg University Hospital with over 40,000 port patients in the past 18 years, port catheters have proven to provide not only the highest quality of life for patients but also a reliable, long-lasting, and safe form of venous access that minimally disrupts daily activities.

This requires skilled and professional port implantation with the correct choice of materials (such as port chamber and catheter sizes), as well as equally professional port care for patients.

1.2 The CVC—Central Venous Catheter

The CVC is by far the most commonly used central venous catheter, employed in acute medicine, intensive care units, and for anesthesia. The preferred sites for access are the internal jugular vein, external jugular vein, and subclavian vein. The femoral vein can also be used for CVC placement when needed. The CVC is usually inserted by venous puncture. The dwell time of a CVC is not clearly defined. VCs should be removed as soon as the indication ceases, as evidence from multiple studies does not support routine replacement for infection prevention (Bundesgesundheitsbl 2017) (Fig. 1.3).

1.3 PICC Catheter

Peripherally inserted central catheters (PICCs) are placed via a peripheral vein, such as the cephalic or basilic vein, through either percutaneous puncture or venous cutdown, and then advanced to a central position. They are particularly popular in the United States (Fig. 1.4). Compared to ports, PICC catheters do have a higher risk of infection, but their outcomes are very close to those of port catheters. However, they have a manufacturer-defined maximum dwell time, which should not exceed three months. The PICC catheter offers a safe temporary alternative to conventional CVCs for medium-term central venous access and support diverse clinical applications Nevertheless, it also carries typical risks inherent to this type of catheter. Displacements of the PICC catheter tip at the atrium of the heart of up to 4 cm

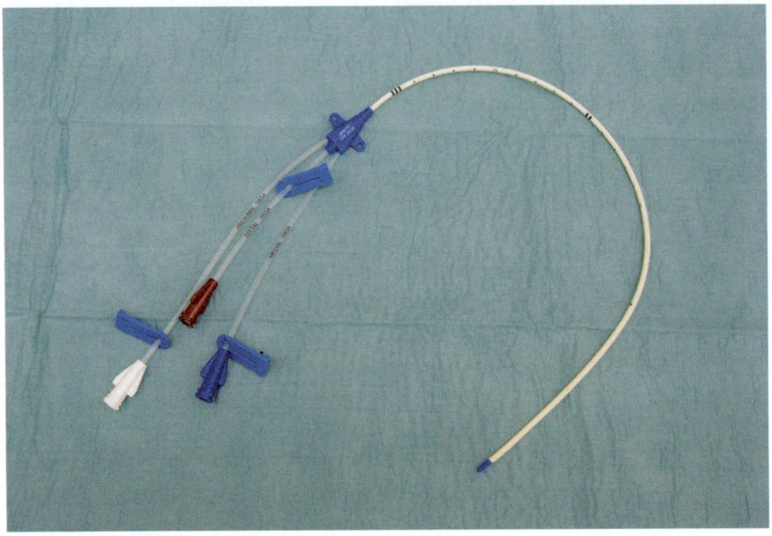

Fig. 1.3 CVC. (© R. Hennes; all rights reserved)

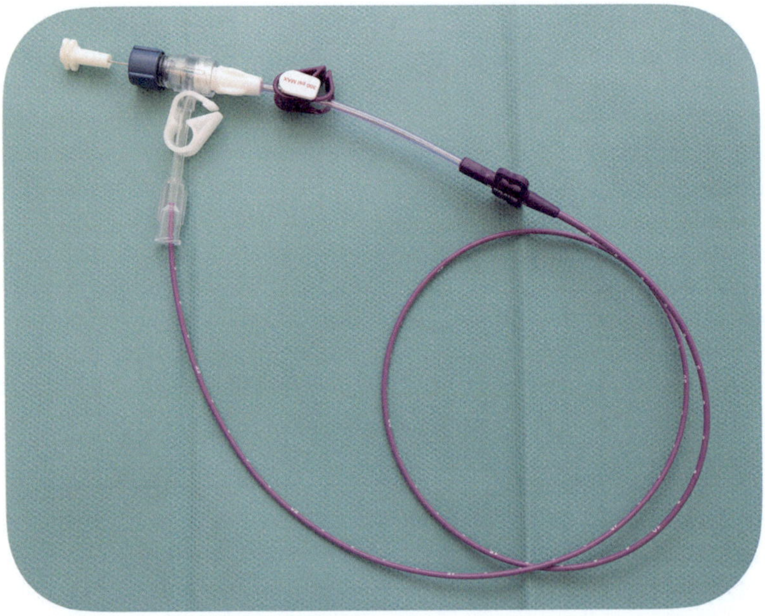

Fig. 1.4 PICC catheter. (© R. Hennes; all rights reserved)

have been observed due to upward movement of the arm and may result incardiac irritationwith arrhythmias that are particularly likely to happen at night (Baskin et al. 2008).

These symptoms can cause significant impairment for patients. In addition, based on our own experience, various mechanical complications of the catheter have been observed, which led to removal of the PICC catheter. These included irritation in the upper arm or catheter fracture with extravasation in the antecubital fossa when placed distally in the forearm (see Chap. 16, Fig. 16.11). Furthermore, patients, especially younger ones, report a reduction in quality of life, due to restrictions such as the inability to swim and limitations on arm use during physical acitivity or exertion.

Several studies have also shown that PICC catheters are associated with significantly increased risks of thrombosis, thrombophlebitis, catheter malposition, and dislocation (Patel et al. 2014; Chopra et al. 2013).

1.4 Hickman Catheter

The Hickman catheter is a partially implanted catheter that can remain in the body for an extended period (over 1 year). Hickman catheters are available in single- and multi-lumen versions. Indications include administration of stem cells, parenteral nutrition, and chemotherapy. As with all catheters, strict adherence to hygiene measures is essential. The catheter is only partially implanted, typically tunneled pectorally, and remains highly susceptible to trauma and rough handling. In clinical practice, it is repeatedly observed that the catheter is accidentally pulled during showering or other personal hygiene activities. The Dacron cuff, which anchors the catheter just beneath the exit site, provides only limited fixation. This should be thoroughly explained to the patient. Even when the catheter is sutured in place, this only provides limited security. As the catheter is made of silicone, it can be damaged by sharp objects or by pinching with fingernails, resulting in leakage. In this context, it is particularly important to note that clamping with a clip on single-lumen Hickman catheters should only be performed in the reinforced section (see Fig. 1.5).

Port Catheter or Hickman Catheter?

In clinical practice, patients often ask: Should I have a Hickman catheter or a port catheter?

Port Catheter
Advantages:

- can remain in the body for over 5 years
- lowest infection rate

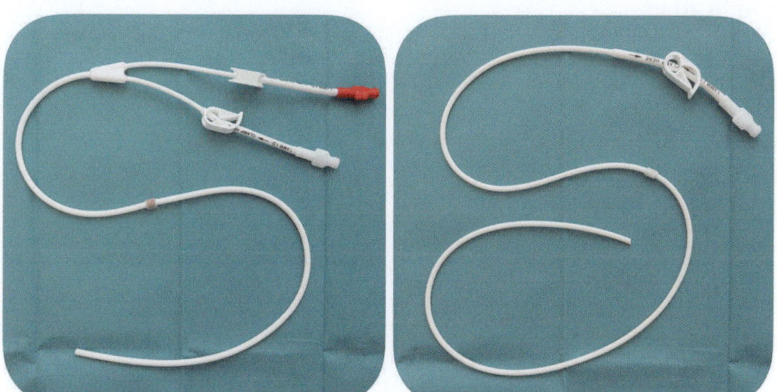

Fig. 1.5 a,b Single- and double-lumen Hickman catheters. (© R. Hennes; all rights reserved)

- best quality of life, no restriction of physical activities

Disadvantages:

- The port chamber must be punctured each time the port catheter is used, or supplied with an indwelling needle for a maximum of 7 days.
- Only trained personnel should care for or access a patient with a port catheter.

Hickman Catheter
Advantages:

- Large volumes can be injected.
- The catheter can also be managed by the patient or relatives after appropriate training.
- Suitable for administration of stem cells.

Disadvantages:

- significant risk of catheter damage
- higher risk of infection
- complex dressing application and changes
- restriction of physical activity and sports

The patient's individual needs should always be the decisive factor in determining the indication.

Case Example
A manager who independently administers his nutritional solution and received training to do so, because he needs to leave for his company early in the morning, insisted on having a Hickman catheter. His priority was his company, not swimming or other athletic pursuits. ◄

1.5 Demers Catheter

The Demers catheter is used for dialysis (Figs. 1.6 and 1.7). Here, only a brief overview of this catheter is provided. For patients, dialysis catheters are of particular importance, as survival and management of impaired renal function are always central concerns. The care and use of the dialysis catheter are exclusively the responsibility of the attending nephrologists and dialysis centers and, especially in the outpatient or home setting, should remain untouched in order to protect the catheter.

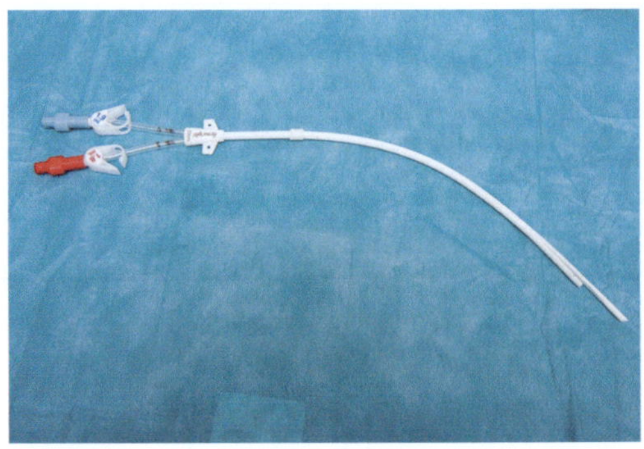

Fig. 1.6 Demers catheter. (© R. Hennes; all rights reserved)

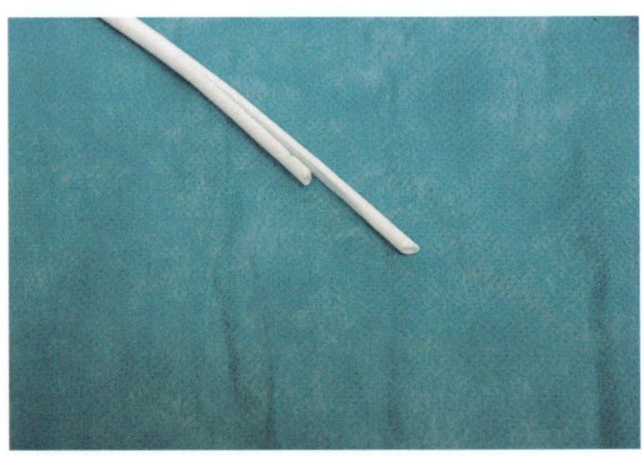

Fig. 1.7 Typical catheter tip of the Demers catheter with different outlets. (© R. Hennes; all rights reserved)

References

Bundesgesundheitsbl (2017) Prävention von Infektionen, die von Gefäßkathetern ausgehen. © Springer-Verlag, Berlin. 60:171–206. https://doi.org/10.1007/s00103-016-2487-4. Zugegriffen: 16. Jan 2017

Baskin KM, Jimenez RM, Cahill AM, Jawad AF, Towbin RB (2008) Cavoatrial junction and central venous anatomy: implications for central venous access tip position. J Vasc Interv Radiol 19(3):359–365. https://doi.org/10.1016/j.jvir.2007.09.005. PMID: 18295694

Chopra V, Anand S, Hickner A et al (2013) Risk of venous thromboembolism associated with peripherally inserted central catheters: a systematic review and meta-analysis. Lancet 382(9889):311–325 22

Chopra V, Anand S, Krein SL, Chenoweth C, Saint S (2012) Bloodstream infection, venous thrombosis, and peripherally inserted central catheters: reappraising the evidence. Am J Med 125(8):733–741 2

Patel GS, Jain K, Kumar R et al (2014) Comparison of peripherally inserted central venous catheters (PICC) versus subcutaneously implanted port-chamber catheters by complication and cost for patients receiving chemotherapy for non-haematological malignancies. Support Care Cancer 22(1):121–128 2

Hennes R, Müller G (2021) Portpflege. Springe. ISBN 978-3-662-60482-3

Needleman J, Buerhaus P, Mattke S, Stewart M, Zelevins ky K (2002) Nurse-staffing levels and the quality of care in hospitals. N Engl J Med 346:1715–1722.

2 Evidence for Port Implantation

Reinhart T. Grundmann

Regarding the question of whether, during the implantation of a port system, the V. cephalica should be surgically exposed ("cutdown") or the catheter should be implanted via puncture of the V. subclavia, a meta-analysis by Klaiber et al. (2021) is available. Based on six randomized studies involving 1,831 patients, the authors concluded that the open technique is significantly superior to the puncture technique in terms of reducing the risk of pneumothorax (odds ratio, OR 0.308; 95% confidence interval, CI 0.122 to 0.776). There were no differences between the two methods with respect to morbidity and mortality. However, the primary failure rate was higher with the open approach (OR 2.364, 95% CI 1.051 to 5.315). Since pneumothorax is a serious complication, the authors advocated for the open approach as the first-line method for the implantation of access ports.

R. T. Grundmann (✉)
Arzt für Chirurgie, Unfallchirurgie, Gefäßchirurgie, Medizinischer Sachverständiger, Burghausen, Germany
e-mail: grundmann@medsachverstand.de

2.1 Meta-analyses and Randomized Studies on Port Implantation

Techniques of Port Implantation
Regarding the implantation of a port system, a meta-analysis by Klaiber et al. (2021) addresses whether surgical exposure ("cutdown") of the cephalic vein or percutaneous cannulation of the subclavian vein is preferable. Based on six randomized studies with 1,831 patients, the authors concluded that open cutdown technique is significantly superior to percutaneous puncture in reducing pneumothorax risk (odds ratio, OR 0.308; 95% confidence interval, CI 0.122 to 0.776). There were no differences between the two methods regarding morbidity and mortality. However, the primary failure rate was higher with the open approach (OR 2.364, 95% CI 1.051 to 5.315). Since pneumothorax is a serious complication, the authors advocated for the open approach as the first-line method for access port implantation. A limitation of this analysis was the variation in techniques used for closed cannulation. The authors concluded that a significantly lower pneumothorax rate (than observed here) might be seen if closed cannulation were consistently performed under ultrasound guidance.

Prior to this analysis, a Cochrane review had been published (Hsu et al. 2016). These authors found moderate quality evidence supporting the statement that the Seldinger technique has a

R. Hennes (ed.), *Port Surgery*, https://doi.org/10.1007/978-3-662-70624-4_2

higher primary implantation success rate compared to venous cutdown.

Moderate quality evidence indicated that, overall, there were no significant differences in complication rates between the Seldinger technique and the open approach. However, when the V. subclavia was used as the access site in the Seldinger technique, the risk of catheter-related complications was higher than with the open approach. These authors found no significant differences in pneumothorax or infection rates between the Seldinger and cutdown groups. The review could not determine which vein would be the optimal access site for the Seldinger technique. In clinical practice, the V. jugularis interna is the most commonly used venous access. In contrast, in the majority of the analyzed studies, the V. subclavia was used as the venous access for the Seldinger technique. The review further stated that the Seldinger technique should always be performed under ultrasound guidance.

Following this Cochrane review, the randomized controlled PORTAS-3 study was published (Hüttner et al. 2020), comparing the open approach versus closed implantation (Seldinger technique). In this study, the primary open approach involved surgical exposure of the V. cephalica. If catheter placement was not possible, the catheter was placed over a guidewire with venous dilation. In the closed technique, the V. subclavia was directly punctured, either using anatomical landmarks, ultrasound guidance, or fluoroscopic control. The study included 1,159 patients (open n = 583; closed n = 576). The rate of pneumothorax or hemothorax was significantly reduced after open port placement (odds ratio 0.27; 95% confidence interval [CI] 0.09–0.88; P = 0.029) (pneumothorax rate with open approach 0.7%, with closed approach 2.5%; hemothorax rate open 0.2%, closed 0.0%). There were no significant differences in 30-day mortality or morbidity. Based on the lower pneumothorax/hemothorax rate, the authors concluded that the open surgical approach should be considered the reference standard technique for port implantation. It should be noted critically that in this study, venous puncture was performed using landmarks for 546 out of 576 patients (94.8%) in the Seldinger group—a technique already described as suboptimal in the Cochrane review (Hsu et al. 2016).

Port vs. Peripherally Inserted Central Venous Catheter for Chemotherapy

In a randomized Swedish two-center study (Taxbro et al. 2019), cancer patients (mainly breast and colorectal) received chemotherapy either via a peripherally inserted central venous catheter (PICC) (n = 201) or via a port (n = 198). The observation period was one year. The PICCs were associated with 16 (8%) deep vein thromboses, compared to 2 (1%) in the port group (p = 0.002). In addition, the incidence of adverse events (composite endpoint) was significantly higher with PICCs than with ports (hazard ratio, HR 2.7; 95% confidence interval 1.6–4.6; P < 01). The authors described their study as the largest randomized trial to date comparing PICCs and ports in cancer patients receiving chemotherapy. The study demonstrated the superiority of port implantation with respect to catheter-related thrombosis and adverse events compared to peripherally inserted PICCs.

Taxbro et al. (2020) also published a cost analysis of their randomized study. In this health economic analysis, placement of a PICC was associated with higher costs compared to port implantation when clinically relevant outcome parameters such as catheter insertion, care, and removal were included. The cost difference was mainly determined by the expenses associated with managing adverse events. When combining costs across all categories, the price for an implanted device was 824.58 EUR for PICCs compared to 662.34 EUR for ports. When costs were adjusted for catheter dwell time, the costs were 6.58 EUR/day for PICCs and 3.01 EUR/day for ports. Thus, from a health economic perspective, the daily costs for PICCs are approximately twice as high as for ports.

The study by Taxbro et al. (2019) ultimately confirms the results of an earlier small randomized study by Patel et al. (2014), in which 70 patients were assigned to either a PICC or a port group for chemotherapy in non-hematological malignancies. In this study, the median dwell time was longer for ports than for PICCs (160 vs. 115 days; p=0.0057), and ports had significantly fewer complications (hazard ratio 0.25, CI 0.09–0.86, P=0.038). Per 100 catheter days, 0.047 major complications were observed after port placement compared to 0.193 after PICC insertion, corresponding to 6% vs. 20% of patients. Thrombosis was the most common complication, occurring in 25% of PICC patients versus 0% in the port group. There were no differences between the groups in terms of quality of life or costs.

Wound Closure after Port Implantation

Witting et al. (2021) included a total of 156 patients with an indication for port implantation in a prospective randomized controlled single-center study. The skin wound was closed either with tissue adhesive or with intracutaneous sutures. Primary endpoints included overall scar assessment by patients and investigators. Secondary endpoints included, among others, complications (inflammation, wound dehiscence) and the duration of wound closure. Patient assessment demonstrated non-inferiority of wound closure with adhesive compared to closure with sutures. Investigators and blinded assessors rated closure with sutures better than closure with adhesive. There were no significant differences between the groups regarding quality of life, wound infection, or dehiscence rates. The authors concluded that sealing the superficial skin layer is a suitable and safe option for wound closure after port implantation.

2.2 Retrospective Studies on Port Implantation

Open Port Implantation via the Jugular Vein Using the Seldinger Technique

Becker et al. (2021) retrospectively analyzed data from 500 consecutive patients who underwent open Seldinger technique port catheter implantation into the jugular vein. The implantation was performed under general or regional anesthesia, with malignancies being the leading indication (in 96.6%). The primary technical success rate was reported as 100%, with an average operative time of 35.9 ± 15.8 (14 to 175) min. Intraoperative complications occurred in 4 cases (0.8%), including one accidental puncture of the carotid artery and one pneumothorax. During the 30-day postoperative follow-up, 4 complications were observed, including one postoperative hemorrhage requiring revision and three wound infections, one of which necessitated port removal. During follow-up of up to one year, 22 infections occurred that required port removal. The cumulative port removal rate after one year was 5.6% (28 cases). The authors described this technique as a safe approach when the conditions for open access via the cephalic vein are not met. Disadvantages included relatively long operative times and a high proportion of procedures performed under general anesthesia (72%).

Closed Port Implantation via the Jugular Vein Using the Seldinger Technique

Tsuruta et al. (2020) reported on long-term outcomes in 482 patients who underwent port implantation via the internal jugular vein using the Seldinger technique. This was a closed procedure with ultrasound-guided puncture of the internal jugular vein, preferably on the right side (88.2%), under local anesthesia. The median observation period for the ports was 319 days, corresponding to 218,971 catheter days. The cumulative port availability was 70% after 3 years. The incidence of complications was 9.1% (0.201 complications/1000 catheter days), and the incidence of infections was 4.4% (0.096 infections/1000 catheter days). The rate of catheter-related complications was reported as 2.9% (0.064/1000 catheter days), and the rate of port-related complications as 1.9% (0.041/1000 catheter days). In this series, patient age < 65 years was associated with a higher complication rate, as was the presence of non-gastrointestinal diseases.

Closed Implantation (Seldinger Technique) Without Ultrasound Guidance

Paprottka et al. (2019) reported a retrospective single-center study of 8,654 radiological port implantations using the Seldinger technique without ultrasound guidance via the subclavian vein. The technical success rate was 99.8%, and the complication rate was 6.52%. Peri-, early, and late complications after the intervention were observed in 1.69%, 0.15%, and 4.68%, respectively. The peri-interventional pneumothorax rate was 1.02%, and arterial punctures/hematomas were seen in 0.34%. The complication rate depended on the interventionalist's level of training, with a pneumothorax rate of 0.5% among experienced physicians versus 1.16% among physicians in training ($p=0.028$), a rate of accidental arterial punctures of 0.12% vs. 0.42% ($p=0.034$), and hematomas of 0.25% vs. 0.35% ($p=0.049$). The authors described their study as the largest retrospective study to date on complications in radiological port implantation and highlighted the low complication rate, even when implantation was performed without ultrasound guidance.

Arm Ports

Xu et al. (2020) reported on more than 570 women with early breast cancer who had a port placed in the upper arm under local anesthesia. Catheter implantation was performed using the Seldinger technique under ultrasound guidance, with puncture of an upper arm vein (basilic or brachial vein). Complications were observed in 32 patients, including one early port removal, corresponding to a complication rate of 0.263/1000 catheter days. Infections ($n=13$) and thromboses ($n=8$) were the most common complications. The authors saw the advantage of their method in avoiding serious complications such as pneumothorax, hemothorax, or arterial punctures. Additionally, for aesthetic reasons, women preferred upper arm port placement over chest wall placement.

For the comparison of arm ports versus chest wall ports, Liu et al. (2020) conducted a systematic review with meta-analysis based on 6 comparative studies and 16 single-arm studies. The specific location of the arm port (upper or lower arm) was not specified. No overall differences in complication rates were found between arm and chest wall ports in the comparative studies. However, when all studies were considered together, the risk of overall complications and catheter-related thromboses may be higher with arm ports. These authors considered chest wall ports to be more suitable than arm ports for women with breast cancer. Given the overall weak evidence base, randomized studies would be necessary to make a definitive statement.

Wildgruber et al. (2015) reported on 1,704 consecutive patients in whom the port catheter was inserted centrally after puncture of the cubital vein, usually via the brachial vein and less frequently via the cephalic vein, with the port itself placed in the forearm. They reported a technical success rate of 99.2% (1,690/1,704 cases) for implantation and a complication rate of 3.2% (55/1,704). The complications were categorized as minor, with no major complications occurring peri-interventionally. The follow-up covered 643,200 catheter days, or 380.6 days per patient. In total, 243 complications (14.4%) were observed in 226 patients (0.4/1000 catheter days), and in 140 patients (8.3%) the port had to be removed. Disconnections between port and catheter were seen in 1.6%, fractures in 0.8%, and leakages in 0.6%. These occurred more frequently when the catheter was inserted via the cephalic vein rather than the brachial vein. Venous thromboses were documented in 40 patients (0.0622/1000 catheter days). The authors described their technique as a minimally invasive approach that avoids major complications (such as pneumothorax). They also stated that forearm port implantation is not associated with an increased rate of thrombosis. Due to the low complication rate, they considered forearm port implantation to be at least equivalent to chest wall ports and possibly superior in terms of patient comfort and cosmetic outcomes.

Deep Vein Thrombosis of the Upper Extremity

The indwelling port catheter, combined with hypercoagulability in some tumors, exposes patients with a port to an increased risk of deep vein thrombosis of the upper extremity (UEDVT). Tabatabaie et al. (2017) investigated risk factors for UEDVT in port patients with the aim of identifying patient groups who might benefit from thrombosis prophylaxis. In this study, 926 of 51,049 patients (1.81%) developed UEDVT, which occurred late (median 95.5 days). In multivariate analysis, age < 65 years, an Elixhauser score of 1 to 2 compared to 0, end-stage renal disease, and a history of DVT were significant predictors of UEDVT. In addition, patients with gastrointestinal cancers, metastases, and lung cancer had a higher risk compared to those with urogenital tumors. Long-term use of antiplatelet agents and/or anticoagulants did not alter the likelihood of UEDVT. The question of whether patients with these risk factors might benefit from thrombosis prophylaxis remained unanswered in this observational study.

Port Fixation

Surgical and interventional textbooks recommend preparing the port pocket down to the level of the pectoral fascia and securing the port there with non-absorbable sutures. This is intended to prevent the port from tipping over or twisting within the pocket during use. Since port fixation may make port removal more difficult, McNulty et al. (2010) omitted preparation of the pectoral fascia and placed the ports in a small subcutaneous pocket without fixation. This involved 534 ports, with a mean port usage duration of 341 days (182,235 port-days). Port tipping occurred in one case (0.2%). Other complications requiring port removal included infections (n=26; 5%), thromboses (n=2; < 1%), catheter fractures (n=1; < 1%), pain (n=2; < 1%), and skin erosions (n=3; 1%). The overall complication rate was 7%. Given that the rate of port tipping in their series was rare and not higher than rates reported in the literature with or without port fixation, the authors continued to advocate against port fixation, as this facilitates port removal and shortens the operative time for port explantation.

Risk of Port Infection and Peri-interventional Antibiotic Prophylaxis

In a retrospective survey by Nezami et al. (2019), 3,978 (67%) of 5,067 patients received perioperative antibiotic prophylaxis during port implantation. Port implantation was performed using the Seldinger technique (mostly via the internal jugular vein) under local anesthesia by a total of 16 interventionalists. In the unmatched population, a total of 65 (1.09%) ports had to be removed within 30 days of placement, 48 of them due to infection or suspected infection (0.27 events/1,000 catheter days). The infection incidence rate was 0.29 events/1,000 catheter days ($n=34$) in patients with antibiotic prophylaxis, compared to 0.24 events/1,000 catheter days ($n=14$) in patients without prophylaxis. The authors also performed propensity score matching with 1,952 patients in each group (antibiotic prophylaxis yes/no). There were no differences between the two groups. In total, 30 ports had to be removed due to infection, 15 in each group, with an infection incidence of 0.26 events/1,000 catheter days. In this survey, the infection rate was significantly higher when the procedure was performed in hospitalized patients compared to outpatient procedures, regardless of antibiotic prophylaxis. The conclusion of this study was that port implantation under inpatient conditions increases the risk of infection. Antibiotic prophylaxis does not reduce the short-term procedure-related infection rate.

The findings of the study by Nezami et al. (2019) are consistent with the results of a previously conducted meta-analysis of four studies involving 2,154 port patients, in which 360 (16.7%) received perioperative antibiotic prophylaxis and 1,794 (83.3%) did not (Johnson et al. 2016). A total of 27 infections (1.25%) were observed, 5 in the prophylaxis group (1.39%) and 22 (1.23%) in the non-prophylaxis group (odds ratio 0.84; CI=0.29–2.35). These authors argued against routine antibiotic prophylaxis during port implantation, although their statements—somewhat ambiguously—seem to focus on radiological port implantation.

Another survey was conducted by Choksi et al. (2020). This study included only radiological procedures (Seldinger technique), in which 709 patients received peri-interventional antibiotic prophylaxis during port implantation, and 752 did not. In this study, 8 ports had to be removed due to infection within 30 days of the procedure, 4 of them in patients with antibiotic prophylaxis (odds ratio 0.97 [95% CI 0.24–3.91; P=0.97; without prophylaxis vs. with prophylaxis]). These authors also did not recommend peri-interventional antibiotic prophylaxis during port implantation.

Time Interval Between Port Placement and Chemotherapy

What influence does the time interval between port placement and the first chemotherapy have on infection rates and port explantation? Kakkos et al. (2017) addressed this question in a prospective observational study involving 4,045 patients. Port implantation was performed either by open or closed technique, most commonly via the internal jugular vein using the Seldinger technique (69.2%). In this series, 7.2% of ports had to be removed due to complications, 2.5% due to infections. There was a significant relationship between the timing of port implantation and the first use of the port. The complication-related port explantation rate was 9.4% when the interval was less than 6 days, compared to 5.7% with an interval of ≥6 days (p=0.008). Another factor influencing the port explantation rate was the leukopenia risk associated with the administered chemotherapy. The port explantation rate due to complications was 5.5% for low and 9.4% for medium or high leukopenia risk (p=0.003). The authors recommended maintaining an interval of 6 days between port implantation and the first chemotherapy to reduce the risk of port explantation due to complications, particularly infections.

Long-term Outcomes After Port Implantation

There are only a few prospective studies that have systematically assessed long-term outcomes after port implantation. One of the largest single-center studies was published by Voog et al. (2018). These authors implanted 493 ports in 483 cancer patients, with a follow-up period ranging from 1 to 94 months (median 18 months), corresponding to a total of 367,359 catheter days. The incidence of complications ($n=87$) was 0.237/1,000 catheter days overall, with few major complications. The infection rate ($n=37$) was calculated at 0.101/1,000 catheter days, and that of symptomatic thromboembolic events ($n=17$) at 0.046/1,000 catheter days. Additionally, 9 cases of extravasation were observed. Of the 87 adverse events, 62 (71.3%) occurred within the first year after implantation; thereafter, adverse events were very rare. Forty-one ports had to be removed due to complications, including 9 due to port infections, 9 due to sepsis, and 9 due to venous thrombosis. The median time to port removal due to a complication was 264 days after implantation (range 8 to 2,533 days). Based on these data, the authors described port tolerance for chemotherapy as excellent.

Port Implantation as a Training Procedure

In the study by Becker et al. (2021), 26.8% of procedures were performed by residents, with no significant differences in complication rates compared to attending physicians. Schreckenbach et al. (2018) also investigated, in a cohort of 760 port implantations, whether outcomes of port implantation (open approach via the cephalic vein) differed depending on whether the procedures were performed by trainees (Group A), trainees assisted by attendings (Group B), or by attending physicians (Group C). There were no significant differences between the groups regarding intraoperative and major postoperative complications. However, operative times differed significantly: Group A averaged 49 min, Group B 53 min, and Group C 39 min. The wound infection rate was 3.6% in Group A versus 0.3% in Group C (p=0.003), and 2.5% versus 0.3% in Groups B versus C (p=0.027). Given that there were no differences in major complications between the groups, the authors considered port implantation to be a safe procedure for surgical training.

Alsfasser et al. (2016) also addressed port implantation as a training procedure. In their study, the interventional puncture technique was used in 1,322 of 1,423 cases (92.9%), with conversion to the open venous cutdown technique in 19 cases (1.4%). A total of 67 (4.7%) early complications occurred, of which 44 (3.1%)

required revision. The most common was iatrogenic pneumothorax at 2.2% ($n = 32$); of these, 26 patients (1.8%) required chest drainage, and 6 patients (0.4%) were managed conservatively. There were a total of 129 (9.1%) late complications of various types, of which 124 (96%) required revision.

Infection was the most common late complication, occurring in 3.9% ($n = 55$) of cases. The rate of early complications was 8.3% in the first year of training, while the other training levels had early complication rates of approximately 5% or less. The average operative time was 39 ± 0.4 min (range: 15–145 min), with a steady decrease from 45 min in the first year of training to 36 min in the fifth year, and an increase among attending and senior physicians to 37 min and 43 min, respectively. The differences in operative times between the first two years of training and the fifth year/attending status were statistically significant ($p < 0.0001$). The conclusion was that, despite the learning curve, complication rates remained low even in the early years of training. The complication rate was independent of the surgeon's level of training; however, the overall and late complication rates decreased with increasing surgical frequency.

Ertel et al. (2017) highlighted the relationship between the individual surgeon's skill and postoperative outcomes in port implantation ("cutdown" of the subclavian, internal jugular, or cephalic vein). In their study of 1,200 port implantations, they observed considerable differences in outcomes among seven surgeons. The chosen surgical technique accounted for a maximum difference of 15 min in operative time and had relatively little impact on the pneumothorax rate or the need to switch to another technique intraoperatively. More decisive were the individual differences in outcomes between surgeons, with operative times differing by up to 37 min. The two surgeons with the longest operative times also had the highest complication rates. The results were not dependent on the surgeon's case volume, leading to the conclusion that the individual surgeon's technique and skill are more important than experience per se for performing the procedure efficiently and with few complications.

2.3 Conclusion for Clinical Practice

1. The open procedure is the first-line approach for the implantation of access ports. In clinical practice, however, the Seldinger technique is very frequently used, with ultrasound-guided puncture of the internal jugular vein being the preferred method.
2. Chemotherapy administered via a port is significantly superior to a peripherally inserted central venous catheter in terms of catheter-related thrombosis and adverse effects. The port is also the more cost-effective alternative.
3. A port catheter can be centrally inserted after puncture of the cubital vein, usually via the brachial vein and less commonly via the cephalic vein, with the port itself placed in the forearm. This minimally invasive approach avoids major complications (such as pneumothorax). Comparative studies of forearm ports versus chest wall ports are lacking.
4. There is no evidence supporting the need for perioperative antibiotic prophylaxis during port implantation, at least when performed using the Seldinger technique.
5. It is recommended to maintain an interval of 6 days between port implantation and the initiation of chemotherapy in order to reduce the risk of port explantation due to complications (especially infections).
6. The skin wound after port implantation can be closed equally well with an intracutaneous suture or tissue adhesive.
7. Retrospective studies show that port implantation is very well suited as a training procedure. However, operative times are significantly longer than with experienced surgeons.

References

Alsfasser G, Neumann A, Klar E, Eisold S (2016) Portimplantation als idealer Ausbildungseingriff – eine Analyse von 1423 Eingriffen [Venous Access Port Implantation is an Ideal Teaching Operation – An Analysis of 1423 Cases]. Zentralbl Chir 141:183–189

Becker F, Wurche LA, Darscht M, Pascher A, Struecker B (2021) Totally implantable venous access port insertion via open Seldinger approach of the internal jugular vein-a retrospective risk stratification of 500 consecutive patients. Langenbecks Arch Surg 406:903–910

Choksi A, Finnegan K, Etezadi V (2020) Does systemic antibiotic prophylaxis prior to the placement of totally implantable venous access devices reduce early infection? A retrospective study of 1485 cases at a large academic institution. Am J Infect Control 48:95–99

Ertel AE, McHenry ZD, Venkatesan VK, Hanseman DJ, Wima K, Hoehn RS, Shah SA, Abbott DE (2017) Surgeon, not technique, defines outcomes after central venous port insertion. J Surg Res 209:220–226

Hüttner FJ, Bruckner T, Hackbusch M et al (2020) Primary open versus closed implantation strategy for totally implantable venous access ports: the multicentre randomized controlled PORTAS-3 trial PORTAS-3 Trial (DRKS 00004900). Ann Surg 272:950–960

Hsu CC, Kwan GN, Evans-Barns H, Rophael JA, van Driel ML (2016) Venous cutdown versus the Seldinger technique for placement of totally implantable venous access ports. Cochrane Database Syst Rev:CD008942

Kakkos A, Bresson L, Hudry D et al (2017) Complication-related removal of totally implantable venous access port systems: does the interval between placement and first use and the neutropenia-inducing potential of chemotherapy regimens influence their incidence? A four-year prospective study of 4045 patients. Eur J Surg Oncol 43:689–695

Klaiber U, Probst P, Hackbusch M, Jensen K, Dörr-Harim C, Hüttner FJ, Hackert T, Diener MK, Büchler MW, Knebel P (2021) Meta-analysis of primary open versus closed cannulation strategy for totally implantable venous access port implantation. Langenbecks Arch Surg 406:587–596

Liu Y, Li LL, Xu L, Feng DD, Cao Y, Mao XY, Zheng J, Jin F, Chen B (2020) Comparison between arm port and chest port for optimal vascular access port in patients with breast cancer: a systematic review and meta-analysis. Biomed Res Int 2020:9082924

McNulty NJ, Perrich KD, Silas AM, Linville RM, Forauer AR (2010) Implantable subcutaneous venous access devices: is port fixation necessary? A review of 534 cases. Cardiovasc Intervent Radiol 33:751–755

Nezami N, Xing M, Groenwald M, Silin D, Kokabi N, Latich I (2019) Risk factors of infection and role of antibiotic prophylaxis in totally implantable venous access port placement: propensity score matching. Cardiovasc Intervent Radiol 42:1302–1310

Paprottka KJ, Voelklein J, Waggershauser T, Reiser MF, Paprottka PM (2019) Retrospective outcome analysis of rates and types of complications after 8654 minimally invasive radiological port implantations via the subclavian vein without ultrasound guidance. Radiol Med 124:926–933

Patel GS, Jain K, Kumar R et al (2014) Comparison of peripherally inserted central venous catheters (PICC) versus subcutaneously implanted port-chamber catheters by complication and cost for patients receiving chemotherapy for non-haematological malignancies. Support Care Cancer 22:121–128

Schreckenbach T, Münch I, El Youzouri H, Bechstein WO, Habbe N (2019) The Safety Level of Total Central Venous Access Port Implantation Performed by Residents. J Surg Educ 76:182–192

Tabatabaie O, Kasumova GG, Kent TS, Eskander MF, Fadayomi AB, Ng SC, Critchlow JF, Tawa NE, Tseng JF (2017) Upper extremity deep venous thrombosis after port insertion: what are the risk factors? Surgery 162:437–444

Taxbro K, Hammarskjöld F, Thelin B, Lewin F, Hagman H, Hanberger H, Berg S (2019) Clinical impact of peripherally inserted central catheters vs implanted port catheters in patients with cancer: an open-label, randomised, two-centre trial. Br J Anaesth 122:734–741

Taxbro K, Hammarskjöld F, Juhlin D, Hagman H, Bernfort L, Berg S (2020) Cost analysis comparison between peripherally inserted central catheters and implanted chest ports in patients with cancer-A health economic evaluation of the PICCPORT trial. Acta Anaesthesiol Scand 64:385–393

Tsuruta S, Goto Y, Miyake H, Nagai H, Yoshioka Y, Yuasa N, Takamizawa J (2020) Late complications associated with totally implantable venous access port implantation via the internal jugular vein. Support Care Cancer 28:2761–2768

Voog E, Campion L, du Rusquec P et al (2018) Totally implantable venous access ports: a prospective long-term study of early and late complications in adult patients with cancer. Support Care Cancer 26:81–89

Wildgruber M, Borgmeyer S, Haller B, Jansen H, Gaa J, Kiechle M, Meier R, Ettl J, Berger H (2015) Short-term and long-term outcome of radiological-guided insertion of central venous access port devices implanted at the forearm: a retrospective monocenter analysis in 1704 patients. Eur Radiol 25:606–616

Witting S, Ingwersen M, Lehmann T et al (2021) Wound closure after port implantation—a randomized controlled trial comparing tissue adhesive and intracutaneous suturing. Dtsch Arztebl Int 118:749–755

Xu H, Chen R, Jiang C, You S, Zhu Q, Li Y, Li S, Zha X, Wang J (2020) Implanting totally implantable venous access ports in the upper arm is feasible and safe for patients with early breast cancer. J Vasc Access 21:609–614

3 Materials for Port Procedures

Hans Haindl

> **Trailer**
> Ports are the method of choice for establishing long-term central venous access.
>
> There is a wide variety of different ports. They differ in terms of materials, design, price, and quality. This chapter provides an overview of the technical features of ports and their impact on performance. To understand their development, the history of ports is also presented. The aim is to enable selection of ports based on quality criteria and to highlight that, in addition to price, there are other important factors to consider when choosing a port.

3.1 The Port

It consists of a small chamber made of metal, plastic, or other materials, has a silicone lid, and is attached to a catheter. However, the situation is more complex than it appears. This becomes clear when we consider that dwell times and complication rates vary considerably among different port catheters. By now, we have gained substantial knowledge about the behavior of various materials, how a port chamber should be constructed, which catheters are preferable, and how best to secure them. The design of port catheter systems has also evolved over the years.

A particular feature, however, is that this development has not necessarily been evolutionary. In fact, it has been observed that the first port catheter systems on the market (NuTech, Pharmacia) were already optimally designed in many respects, as later comparisons with other port catheter systems have shown. The port catheters introduced more recently have not shown consistent improvement; in fact, many are markedly inferior to the earliest models. This decline largely stems from the continuous drive to produce devices more cost-effectively.

For users, it is difficult to determine whether a higher price actually indicates a better product. For shorter periods of use, one might even say: we do not need the best product; the cheapest one will suffice. The purpose of this chapter is not to prescribe which port should be used, as any such recommendation would represent only a momentary view and would inevitably change with the advent of new products. Rather, this chapter is intended to show you which materials and design features lead to which properties in port catheters, so that you can make a more informed selection.

Compliance with the requirements of DIN EN ISO 10555-6:2020-02 should be a matter of course for every port.

H. Haindl (✉)
Sachverständiger für Medizintechnik, Wennigsen, Germany
e-mail: post@haindl.eu

R. Hennes (ed.), *Port Surgery*, https://doi.org/10.1007/978-3-662-70624-4_3

Statements and illustrations without a source reference are based on our own investigations.

3.2 History

The port catheter is a spin-off that emerged with the introduction of a new technology. The problems and risks associated with externally tunneled vena cava catheters had been known for many years, but no solution had been found. It was only with the development of implantable pumps—and the associated challenge of refilling the pump while it was implanted—that the idea arose to incorporate a silicone septum into the pump, which could be punctured through the skin to refill it. The implantable pumps themselves were a spin-off from aerospace technology (or so the story goes), where a gas propulsion system using a two-phase mixture, similar to that used in implantable pumps, was employed to deliver lubricants to moving parts. The concept of the pump was first described by Blackshear (1970). The first use in animals occurred in 1975, and in humans in 1977. At that time, the primary goal was the continuous administration of heparin. In 1981, the first Infusaid pump received FDA approval.

Infusaid, the first manufacturer of implantable pumps, quickly realized that patients could use a port not only for refilling the pump but also for bolus injections. To this end, a bolus port was added to the Infusaid pump (Fig. 3.1), and at the same time, the Infuse-a-port, a standalone port catheter, was developed (Fig. 3.2). In parallel, several former employees of Infusaid Inc. began developing the Port-a-Cath (Fig. 3.3), which they evidently designed more successfully than the Infuse-a-port, as it is still available today with only minor modifications, whereas the Infusaid port is long gone. It remains unclear who was truly first. The first publication on the Infuse-a-port was by Niederhuber and Ensminger (1982), while the first publication on the Port-a-Cath by NuTech (later Pharmacia) was by Ecoff et al. in (1983).

In parallel with the development of pumps and the resulting ports, Pudenz-Schulte Medical Inc., founded in 1978, also developed an implanted port, but not for drug injection—instead, it was intended for tapping fluid in cases

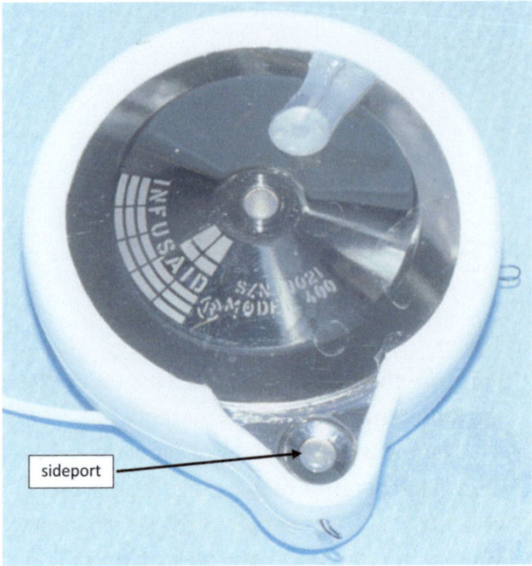

Fig. 3.1 Infusaid pump with side port

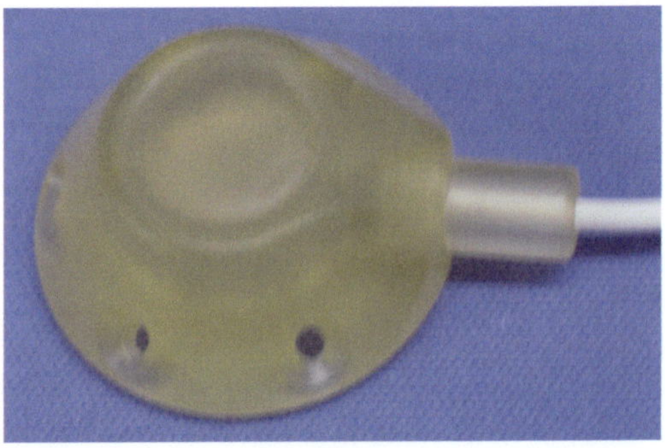

Fig. 3.2 Infuse-a-port by Infusaid

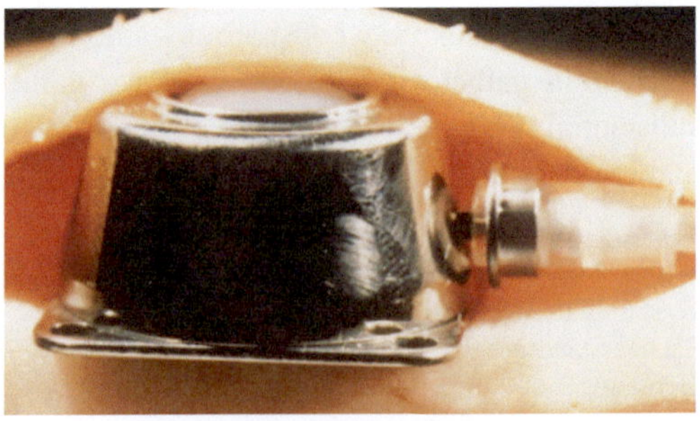

Fig. 3.3 Port-a-Cath by NuTech (later Pharmacia). (Copyright: Rainer Janßen; with kind permission)

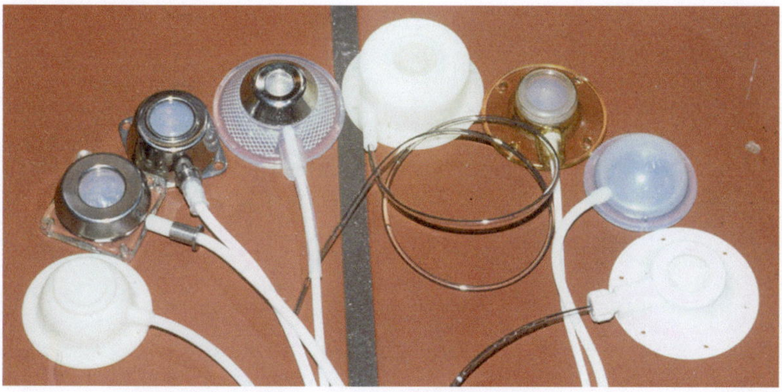

Fig. 3.4 The early port catheters, from left: Vygon Silicon, Baxter, Port-a-cath, Norport, Medinorm, Fresenius Intraport I, Pudenz-Schulte, Braun Implantofix II

of hydrocephalus. This product also had a brief career as a port for drug administration, but it soon became clear that it was not suitable for this purpose. A wide range of products quickly emerged, some of which are shown in Fig. 3.4. From left to right, these are Vygon Silicon, Baxter, Port-a-cath, Norport, Medinorm, Fresenius Intraport I, Pudenz-Schulte, Braun Implantofix II—all of which have since disappeared from the market.

After ports had initially been developed with varying degrees of success in many places, the first publications on the systematic investigation of port properties appeared (Haindl 1989; Janßen 1989), and subsequently, some ports disappeared from the market.

As a special variant of the port catheter, arm ports have occasionally been offered. Pharmacia has a commercially available arm port that is punctured in the conventional manner, i.e., vertically from above. Because it must be constructed to be very flat, it has only a relatively thin membrane and therefore a very limited service life (Fig. 3.5). Fresenius marketed a microport that can be implanted entirely by puncture, but must then be accessed tangentially (Fig. 3.6). There have been many attempts to establish port catheters that must or can be accessed tangentially, but all have been unsuccessful. Apparently, vertical access to the port has become so ingrained in user practice that a change is no longer feasible.

An exception is made for ports used in hemodialysis, where a straight flow path is desirable due to the high blood flow rates (Fig. 3.7). However, these ports have not yet gained widespread acceptance in dialysis.

There have been various attempts to challenge the role of port catheters as long-term central venous access devices. However, their superiority over Hickman and Broviac catheters (Fig. 3.8) has long been established (Ng et al. 2007). In particular, the vulnerability of silicone catheters and the risk of air embolism argue against percutaneous catheters.

A more recent development is the so-called PICC catheter. These are catheters inserted by puncturing a vein in the antecubital fossa or upper arm and advanced to the vicinity of the atrium. It has been shown that these catheters are better tolerated than the earlier basilic catheters, especially when they are placed proximal to the elbow, thereby avoiding irritation of the veins caused by movement in the elbow region. PICC catheters may represent an alternative to ports for shorter indwelling times (Patel et al. 2014).

However, it must not be forgotten that this reintroduces risks that have been successfully avoided with port catheters, particularly the risk of air embolism. The fact that PICC catheters are now often equipped with disinfectable, needleless injection connectors, making accidental air entry after opening the connector

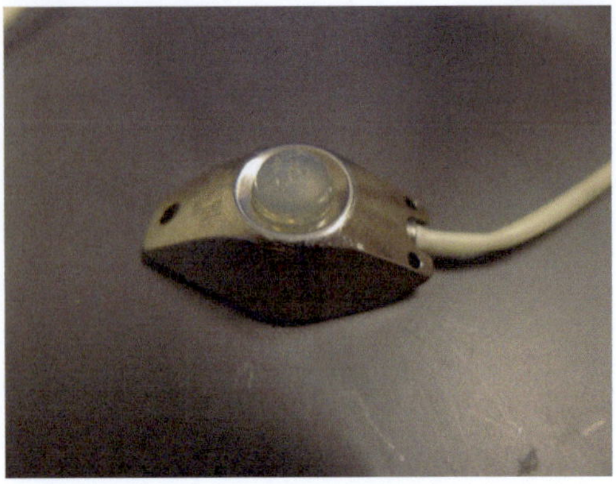

Fig. 3.5 Pharmacia arm port

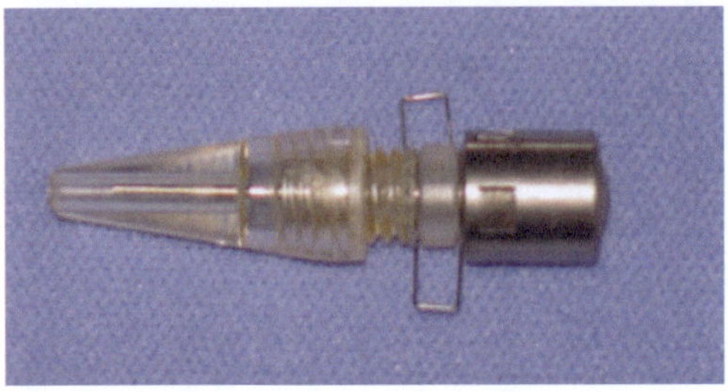

Fig. 3.6 Fresenius microport

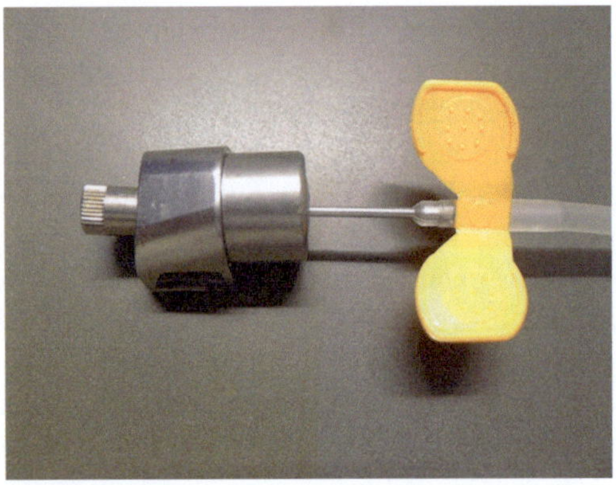

Fig. 3.7 Dialysis port

virtually impossible even without a three-way stopcock, does not change this. Catheter damage must also always be considered, as it is known to occur occasionally, especially during dressing changes. Therefore, the PICC catheter cannot be regarded as a fully equivalent and long-term alternative to the port catheter.

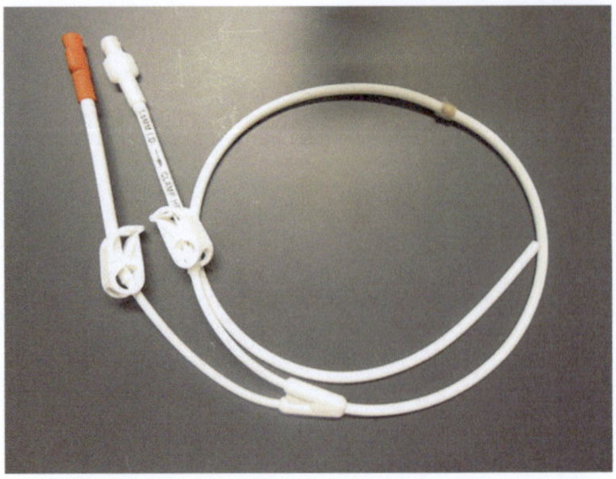

Fig. 3.8 Hickman catheter

3.3 Development

From the very beginning, the team at NuTech led by Elton Tucker understood something that most other port developers overlooked. A high degree of axial compression of the membrane is required to ensure reliable closure even after numerous punctures. We were able to confirm this through simple experiments using a port housing with adjustable membrane tension. In the meantime, many unusual products had appeared on the market, such as a silicone port that could be inflated to many times its original volume with little effort (Fig. 3.9), as well as the Pudenz-Schulte port (Fig. 3.10). Ports with radially compressed membranes were also introduced, but these could not match the service life of the NuTech or Pharmacia ports.

It was evident from the Pharmacia ports that the membrane was under significant pressure. However, for many port manufacturers, plastic was the preferred housing material, and with this material it was difficult to achieve the necessary pressure to compress the membrane to a degree comparable to that of the Pharmacia port. As a workaround, many manufacturers simply simulated the bulging of the membrane under pressure by using injection-molded membranes that produced a pronounced dome over the port even without any pressure (Fig. 3.11).

As ports became more widely used, complications inevitably arose. Occasionally,

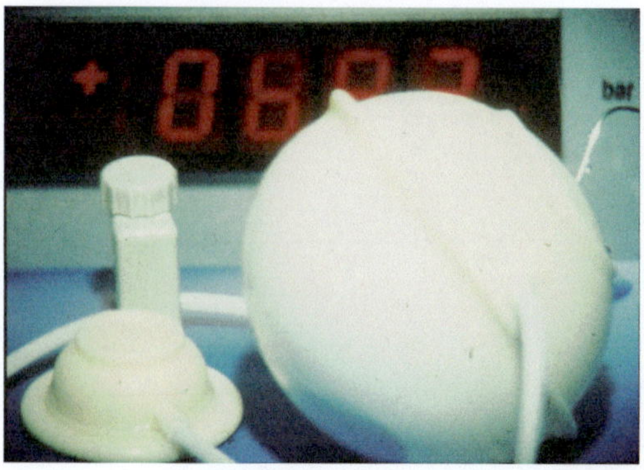

Fig. 3.9 Vygon silicone port

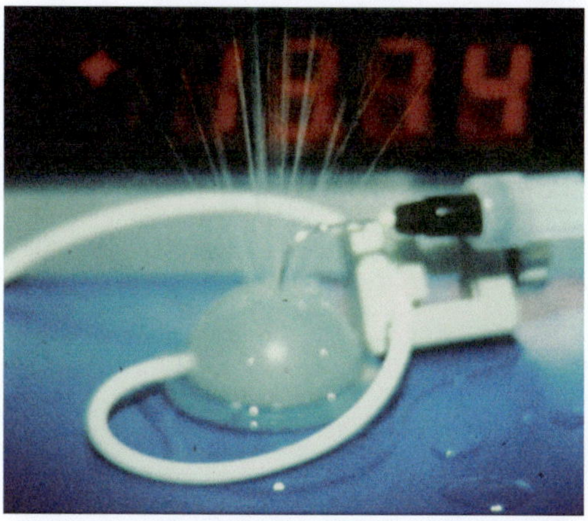

Fig. 3.10 Pudenz-Schulte port

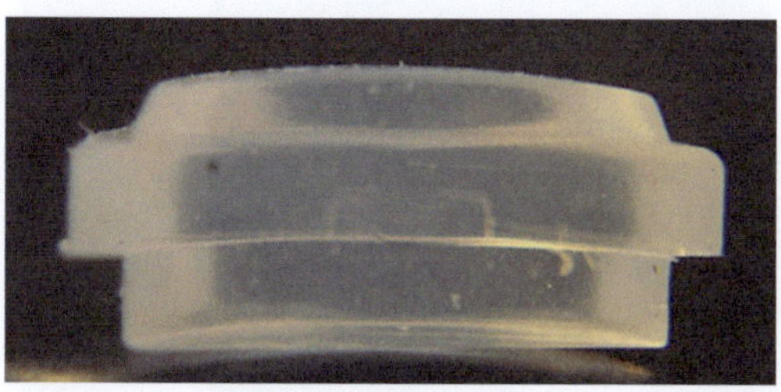

Fig. 3.11 Domed membrane

catastrophic destruction of the membranes occurred (Figs. 3.12 and 3.13), which could be easily explained once the behavior of the needles in the membranes was systematically investigated. It was found that the Huber needle, considered the gold standard of non-coring needles, actually punched out large pieces of the membrane (Müller and Zierski 1988) (Fig. 3.14). The claim of being non-coring had been accepted without question, but apparently no one had ever verified it. This made it clear that the port and needle form a system, and even a high-quality port can only tolerate a poor needle to a limited extent.

Other complications included perforations of port catheters, which were rare but tended to occur during the infusion of cytostatic agents and could lead to significant tissue necrosis (Sharp, Nicole et al. 2014). Perforations occurred mainly in ports made of POM (polyoxymethylene), which has only limited stability in acidic pH environments. Since some cytostatic agents are stabilized in acidic conditions, these may have contributed to the damage. However, we were unable to reproduce the course of damage in the laboratory.

It also became apparent that when the port catheter is used for infusion—when the needle remains in the port for several days and moves within the port due to the patient's body movements—visible material abrasion occurs in plastic ports. Even if this did not always lead to immediate perforation, it became clear that it is undesirable for the resulting particles to end up in the patient's lungs.

This led to a shift toward titanium as a material, since stainless steel proved to be disadvantageous in several respects—not only because of its weight, but also due to pronounced artifacts in cross-sectional imaging. Not everyone was able to process titanium. Because titanium is an expensive material, there were also many attempts to combine materials, for example by incorporating titanium cups or plates into plastic port catheters (Fig. 3.15). Around 1990, aluminum oxide ceramic was introduced as a port material (Fig. 3.16). This material offers several advantages over all other port materials (Haindl et al. 1995), but its high cost prevented widespread adoption.

The last major innovation in the field of port catheters was the development of high-pressure-resistant ports, designed for use with high-pressure injectors for CT-synchronized contrast agent injection at rates of up to 5 ml/s. This was not a true innovation, as some ports on

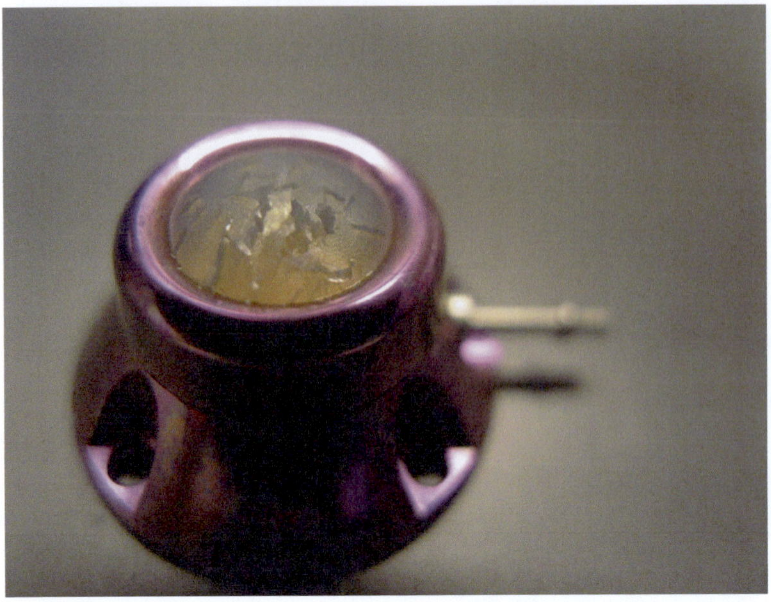

Fig. 3.12 Destroyed membrane

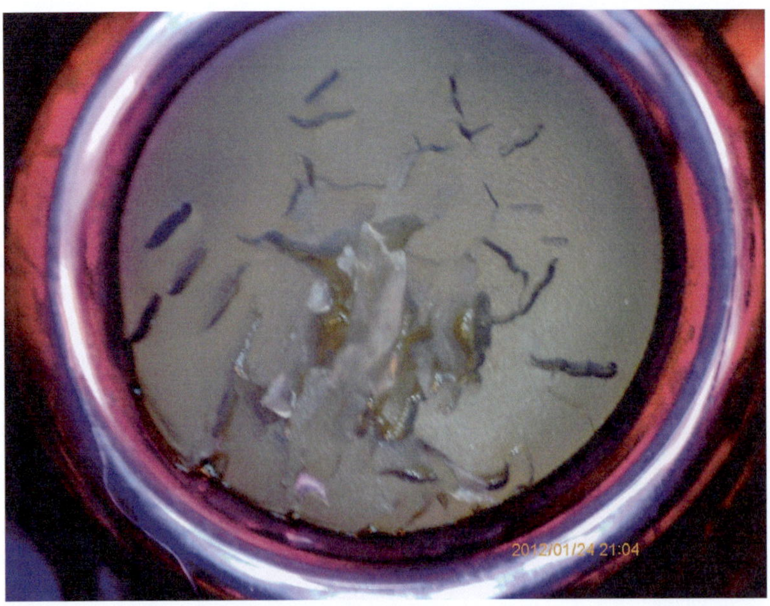

Fig. 3.13 Large puncture scars and extruding silicone

the market already met the pressure resistance requirements at that time. The main novelty was making this feature visible on X-ray images by introducing radiopaque markers into the ports, allowing radiologists to identify ports suitable for high-pressure injection. Since confusion can lead to serious patient injury, it would be desirable for all ports to be suitable for high-pressure injection in the future, which would not pose a technical challenge.

Implantable pumps have also been further developed over time and are mainly used for

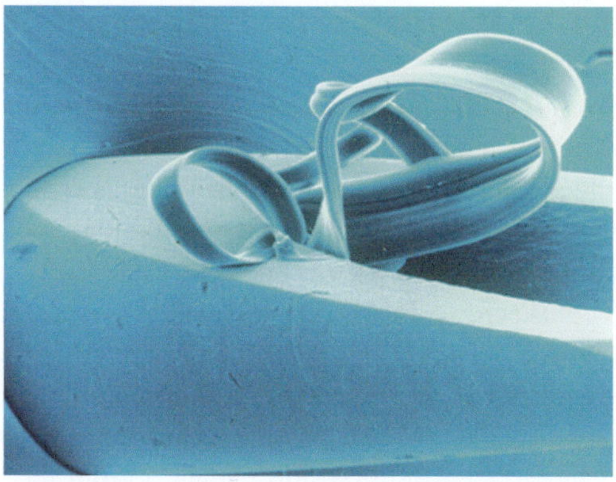

Fig. 3.14 Huber needle after membrane passage

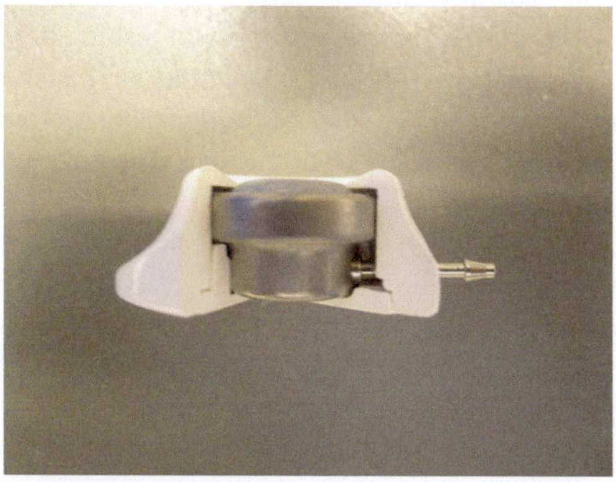

Fig. 3.15 Titanium cup in plastic housing (Braun)

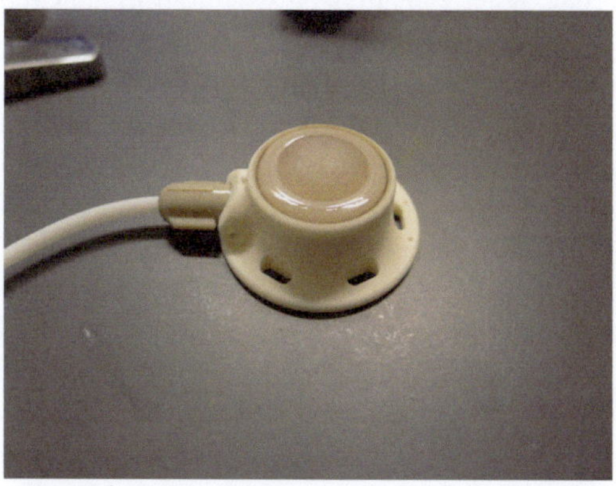

Fig. 3.16 Ceramic port (Fresenius)

continuous intravenous administration of 5-FU in oncology or for the administration of baclofen in the treatment of spasticity, and more recently for the treatment of pulmonary hypertension. In addition to gas pressure-driven pumps, electrically operated pumps that can be controlled externally have also been introduced, and the latest development is gas pressure-driven pumps with electronically controlled settings. As a result, these pumps require significantly less energy, since the pumping function is powered by gas pressure and only a small amount of energy is needed to control the function.

3.4 Technical Challenges in Materials and Design

3.4.1 Construction of the Port Housing

Key design features, such as membrane compression, have already been discussed in Chapter 3, Development. In port construction, there is a conflict between achieving a low profile—which is important for slim or cachectic patients to prevent skin necrosis over the port—and ensuring the port chamber is tall enough to fully accommodate the beveled eye of the port needle. If the port chamber is made too shallow in an effort to reduce the overall height, the beveled eye of the needle may not be completely exposed when the needle tip reaches the chamber floor, further restricting flow, for which the needle is already the limiting factor.

Another effect to consider occurs particularly when the membrane is not sufficiently compressed. In this case, the needle can push the membrane slightly into the port until it contacts the chamber floor. Once the needle is released, the membrane springs back, lifting the needle tip slightly off the chamber floor. This distance must be taken into account when determining the height of the port chamber. The volume of the port chamber varies significantly between different ports. This information, including the catheter volume, should always be communicated to the user to ensure that solutions used to fill the port when not in use can be dosed appropriately.

The joining technique is particularly demanding for plastic ports that need to be pressure-resistant. Snap-fit connections have evidently been abandoned. Ultrasonic welding of the upper and lower port components is also technically challenging due to the intervening silicone membrane. Silicone membranes, which typically have slight variations in thickness, dampen the ultrasonic energy depending on their compression. The design must ensure absolutely reliable welding.

There are numerous variations in the external shape of ports. It is generally true that oval shapes can be more easily inserted through a small skin incision than round ports, but ultimately this is largely a matter of preference. What is important is that the port does not create large cavities in the tissue; it should have as continuous a transition as possible from the top to the bottom so that the tissue can conform well to the device.

A special form is the double-chamber port (Fig. 3.17), which is connected to a dual-lumen catheter. This allows for the simultaneous infusion of substances that are not compatible with each other. However, to truly meet this requirement, it is important that the exit openings at the catheter tip are spaced apart so that the fluids do not come into contact with each other before mixing with blood. If it is possible to infuse the two incompatible agents sequentially, a double-chamber port is not indicated.

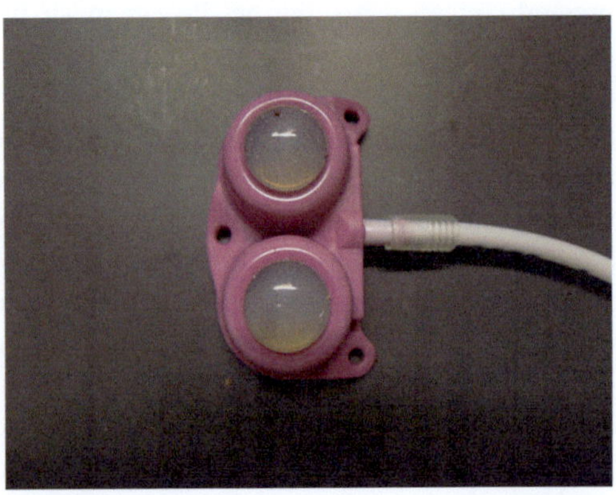

Fig. 3.17 Double-chamber port

3.4.2 Materials of the Port Housing

Even the first port catheters were based on two different approaches. Infusaid produced its port catheters from the plastic polysulfone, accepting that significant membrane compression could not be achieved with this material.

NuTech, or Pharmacia, evidently recognized that the service life of the membrane could be significantly improved by axial compression, and in order to achieve the necessary forces, manufactured the first port catheters from medical-grade stainless steel.

However, due to the high weight of stainless steel, port migration occurred if the device was not absolutely securely fixed. As a result, after a few years, titanium was adopted as the material of choice, and it remains a well-established and effective port material to this day. The only real disadvantage of titanium is that, when used in larger quantities, it causes significant artifacts in CT imaging. For this reason, and also to save on expensive material, many manufacturers have switched over time to combining titanium with plastics—a sensible solution, provided the titanium absorbs the compression forces.

Among plastics, in addition to polysulfone, polyoxymethylene was one of the first materials used for ports. Due to its good spring properties, polyoxymethylene was used to construct port catheters held together by a snap-fit connection (Fig. 3.18). For reasons never fully clarified, some patients experienced disconnection of these snap-fit joints. In addition, during cytostatic therapy, some cases of port chamber floor perforation occurred, probably due to insufficient acid resistance of polyoxymethylene, although this was also never fully explained.

As a result, some manufacturers discontinued the use of polyoxymethylene as a port material, while others continue to use it to this day. Polysulfone has proven to be a reasonably effective port material, even though it does not allow for the desired membrane compression. Over time, it was also observed that, during infusion via the port when the needle remains in place for several days, the needle tip can cause significant particle release from the polysulfone.

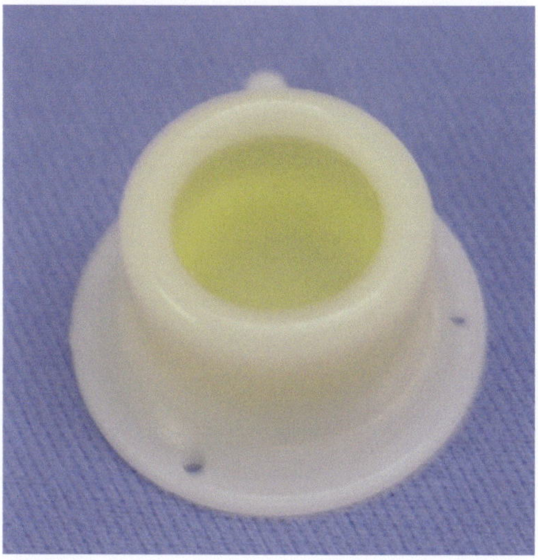

Fig. 3.18 Port with snap-fit housing (Implantofix 1, Braun)

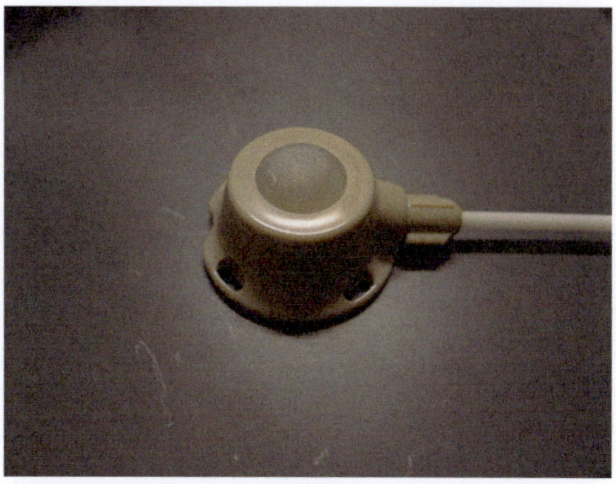

Fig. 3.19 Port made of PEEK (Fresenius)

Attempts have been made, for example using fiber-reinforced materials, to overcome the disadvantages of plastics with respect to membrane compression, but none have been entirely satisfactory. Only with the use of the high-performance plastic PEEK (polyetheretherketone) was it possible to compress the membranes in plastic ports sufficiently to ensure long service life (Fig. 3.19). However, this largely eliminated the cost advantage of plastic ports compared to, for example, titanium ports.

In addition, since 1990, ports made of aluminum oxide ceramic have been available (Fig. 3.16). This material had already proven itself millions of times as an implant material in hip joint prostheses. As a port material, it offered the advantage of not producing any fragmentation and, despite being radiopaque, did not cause artifacts in cross-sectional imaging. However, the relatively high material cost and the demanding joining technique meant that these port catheters, due to their price, only achieved limited distribution. Table 3.1 summarizes the advantages and disadvantages of the various port housing materials.

A distinction is made between conventional plastics, such as polysulfone and polyoxymethylene, on the one hand, and high-performance plastics, such as PEEK, on the other. Both titanium and ceramic are used to reinforce the port bases or the entire inner wall of the port; in some cases, titanium sheet is also used to compress the membrane, while the outer surface of the port is then made of plastic.

Since it is often difficult to combine all the desired properties in a single material in a cost-effective manner, composite designs that combine different materials are increasingly being used.

3.4.3 Catheter Materials

To date, both silicone and polyurethane catheters have proven effective and are used alongside each other. Silicone catheters tend to be preferred when the catheter is inserted into the cephalic vein via cutdown. Polyurethane catheters, on the other hand, are generally favored for port catheter placement via puncture of the subclavian vein or other vessels, as they are easier to advance.

For silicone catheters, the standard material corresponds to Dow Corning material RX 80 with 20% barium sulfate. Since Dow Corning has significantly reduced its activities in the implant business due to negative experiences, this material is now supplied by various other manufacturers. However, these are essentially similar materials, albeit of varying quality.

Table 3.1 Advantages and disadvantages of different port materials

	Steel	Titanium	Plastic e.g., POM/PSU	High-performance plastic e.g., PEEK	Al_2O_3 ceramic
Weight	–	+	+++	+++	+
Scratch resistance/particle formation[3]	++	++	–	+	+++
Membrane compression[3.1]	+++	+++	–/+	+++	+++
Corrosion resistance	+	++	–/+	+++	+++
Artifact-free imaging	–	+	+++	+++	+++
MR compatibility	–	+	+++	+++	+++
Hyperthermia compatibility	–	–	+++	+++	+++
Wettability	–	–	–	–	++
Damage to cannula tip[2]	–	–	++	+	–
High-pressure resistance	+++	+++	–/++	+++	+++

[1] Membrane compression is crucial for the stability of the membrane and the pressure resistance of the port. The achievable membrane compression varies greatly depending on the type of plastic.
[2] The decisive factor here is the material of the port base.
[3] There is a trade-off between the scratch resistance of the port base and the risk of damage to the cannula tip: the better the scratch resistance, the greater the risk of damage to the cannula tip.

The excellent long-term durability of silicone, which was primarily recognized through experience with silicone breast implants, unfortunately cannot be directly transferred to the situation with port catheters. The addition of barium sulfate to make the catheter radiopaque affects its long-term stability. During explantation of port catheters that have been in place for a long time (over five years), it is often found that the material has lost its tensile strength and breaks under even slight tension. Therefore, it appears advisable to limit the duration of implantation.

Another issue is that different grades of silicone used for tubing manufacture exhibit varying strengths. For example, we observed significant fluctuations in burst pressure among silicone tubes with identical inner and outer diameters, ranging from 400 to 900 kPa.

Similar problems regarding long-term stability have been reported for polyurethanes.

Very good experience has been gained with the aliphatic polyurethane elastomer Tecoflex in central venous catheters, as it becomes softer within blood vessels. As a result, many port catheter manufacturers have used this material for port catheter tubing. However, this has led to problems for some manufacturers. Tecoflex is susceptible to stress cracking. It demonstrates excellent long-term stability in the human body as long as it is not under tension.

Some port catheter manufacturers have used cannulas with olive-shaped expansions for port couplings, which have stretched the Tecoflex catheters circumferentially by more than 100%. In such cases, tearing, stress cracking, and pitting of the plastic have occurred (Figs. 3.20 and 3.21). Provided that such stress-inducing measures are avoided, Tecoflex appears to be sufficiently stable for periods of around five years.

Alternatively, polycarbonate urethanes such as Chronoflex or Carbothane are recommended, as they offer significantly better long-term stability.

3.4.4 Membranes

The membranes for port catheters are all made of silicone rubber. The decisive factors for this choice are, on the one hand, the high elasticity and resulting excellent resealing capability, and on the other hand, the inert behavior of the material as an implant.

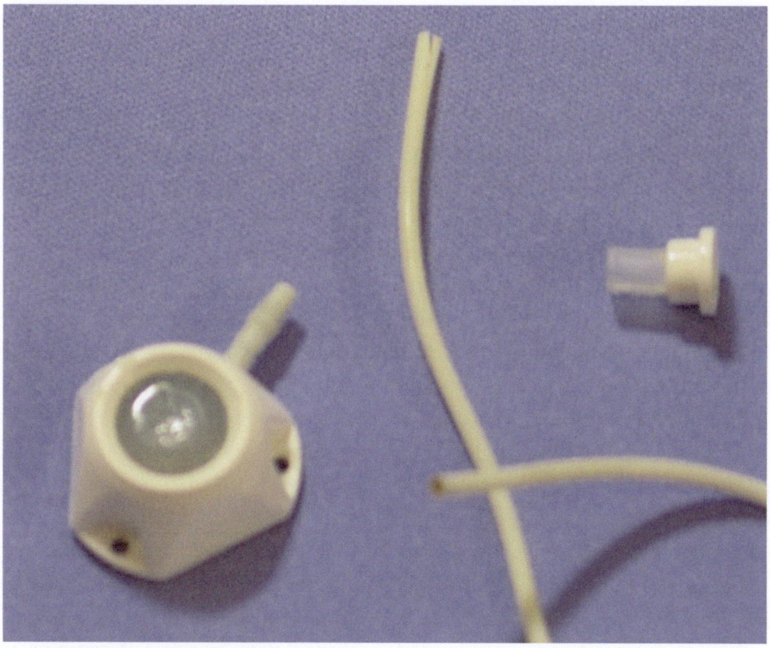

Fig. 3.20 Catheter torn off at the support cannula

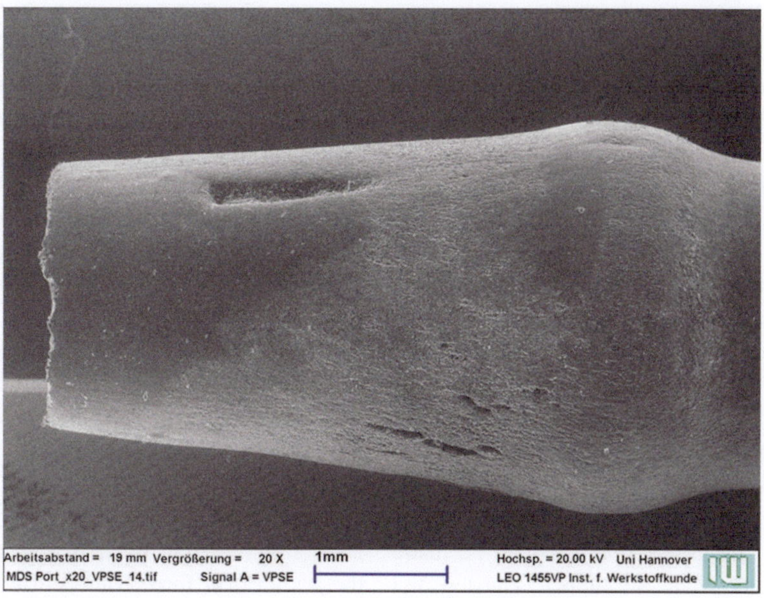

Fig. 3.21 SEM image 20x: stress cracks and pitting

However, not all silicone membranes are the same. Essentially, two different groups of silicones are used. One group comprises so-called liquid silicone rubbers (LSR), which are mixed from two components and can be processed by injection molding. These materials have the advantage of very simple processing, allowing even complex shapes. However, they are rarely used for port catheters.

The so-called high consistency silicone rubbers are preferable; these are usually platinum-cured for use in implants. The manufacturing process is complex. The liquid to pasty starting material must be mixed with the catalyst, then repeatedly calendered for pre-polymerization to form a gel-like, plastically deformable intermediate product. This intermediate product can then be portioned by weight or volume and placed into a compression mold, where it is hot-pressed.

For higher production volumes, so-called injection compression molding can also be used, in which portioning is performed within the machine and is volumetrically controlled. Among these high consistency rubbers, there is a subgroup known as ETR silicones (Extended Tear Resistance). These materials have nearly double the elongation at break compared to LSR silicones and, in particular, exhibit very high tear propagation resistance. This property is especially important for use as a port membrane.

The resealing properties of the membrane are particularly good when it is also clamped under pressure. The axial compression of the membrane edge, as used in the first port by NuTech, has proven especially effective. This significantly increases the resealing capability, as it greatly reduces the particle punching effect, which is most pronounced at the membrane surface. Of course, this always requires the use of suitable needles.

However, the clamping of the membrane can also be achieved in different ways. The diameters of the clamping housing components can be the same above and below the membrane. Alternatively, the lower diameter can be made slightly smaller than the upper, causing the membrane to bulge more upwards rather than into the port. This appears to be a favorable clamping method. If the opposite is done, i.e., the upper clamping diameter is smaller than the lower, the risk of hitting the lower compression edge when puncturing the membrane is reduced, but the disadvantage is that the bulging of the membrane is mainly directed into the port interior, thereby reducing the usable height of the port chamber.

A good port can thus be recognized by the fact that the membrane protrudes slightly upwards and is relatively firm because it is pre-tensioned.

Of course, it is possible to take a very simple approach by injection-molding a membrane from LSR silicone that is convex on the upper surface from the outset (Fig. 3.11). The port then looks just as attractive, but its resealing performance falls far short of that of a well-designed port. The performance differences resulting from material selection and membrane clamping are considerable.

The initial claims by manufacturers of leak-tightness after more than 2,000 punctures are rather optimistic. A port can already be considered very good if it remains leak-tight after approximately 1,000 punctures with a 22 G port needle. However, it is not uncommon for port catheter systems to become leaky much earlier, for example after about 200 punctures, even when good port needles are used.

Systems with a stepped membrane (Fig. 3.11), in which the clamping occurs only over a reduced membrane thickness, may become leaky after just a few punctures at the membrane edge if the punctures are unfortunately placed. Port catheters that look identical may differ by a factor of four or more in terms of the number of possible punctures.

Another property related to the membrane and its clamping is the insertion force and withdrawal force of the port needles. Ideally, a port needle would be easy to insert but would then sit firmly and be difficult to withdraw. Unfortunately, this combination is not achievable. The insertion force is always higher than the withdrawal force. Here, different properties must be weighed against each other.

A high insertion force means that more force is required to insert the needle, and the needle tip, under this force, may strike the port base. This leads to increased tip damage and, consequently, to membrane damage when the needle is withdrawn. In this respect, a high insertion force is rather disadvantageous. The situation is different with withdrawal force. Here, it would of course be desirable for it to be somewhat higher; on the other hand, the relative disadvantage of reduced withdrawal force can be compensated for by an appropriate needle fixation system.

3.4.5 Catheter Couplings

While disconnections and catheter breakages at the port catheter coupling have become rare today, this was not always the case. The first port catheter couplings essentially consisted of a cannula onto which the tube was pushed, and a sleeve that was slid over it. The diameter of the sleeve was such that it could still be moved, but pressed the port catheter relatively firmly onto the cannula. When such couplings are tested in the laboratory, the measured holding strengths exceed the tensile strength of the tubing material. Nevertheless, this type of port catheter coupling repeatedly led to disconnections (Fig. 3.20).

There is a trade-off between the secure mechanical clamping of the catheter onto the support cannula and the strength and corrosion resistance of the catheter material. The more the tubing material is bent and thus stretched, for example over an olive, the better it holds on the support cannula. At the same time, however, the strong stretching of the material reduces the tensile strength of the tube, and certain materials may also develop corrosion phenomena (stress corrosion). In silicone tubes, the silicone may also be crushed on the olive (Fig. 3.22).

When different types of support cannulas are viewed side by side, it becomes apparent that not all port manufacturers are aware of this relationship (Fig. 3.23).

The misuse safety of the couplings must also be considered. Frequently, the catheters must be pushed onto a support cannula up to a specific point before the coupling is closed.

3.4.6 Port Needles

As early as 1988, Müller and Zierski (1988) pointed out that commercially available Huber needles do not always fulfill their promise of being non-coring. This is because Huber's idea—to bend the needle tip so that the rear bevel eye is essentially placed in the shadow of the tip—may seem plausible at first glance,

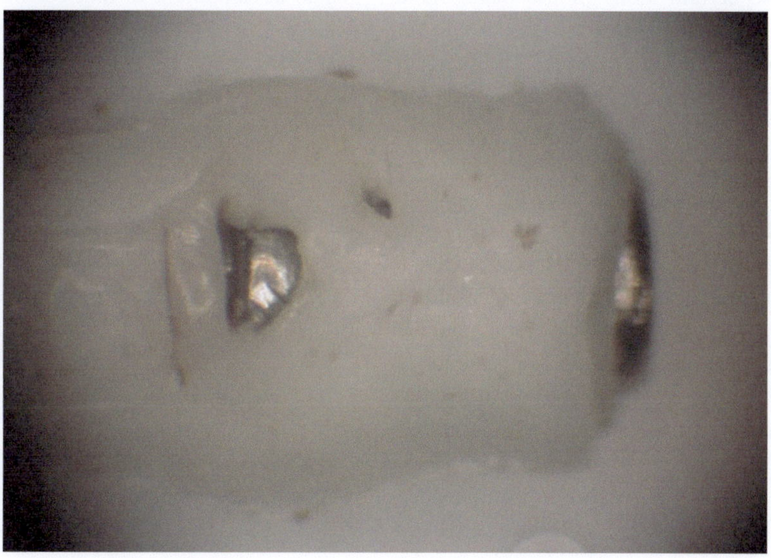

Fig. 3.22 Silicone tube crushed on the coupling olive

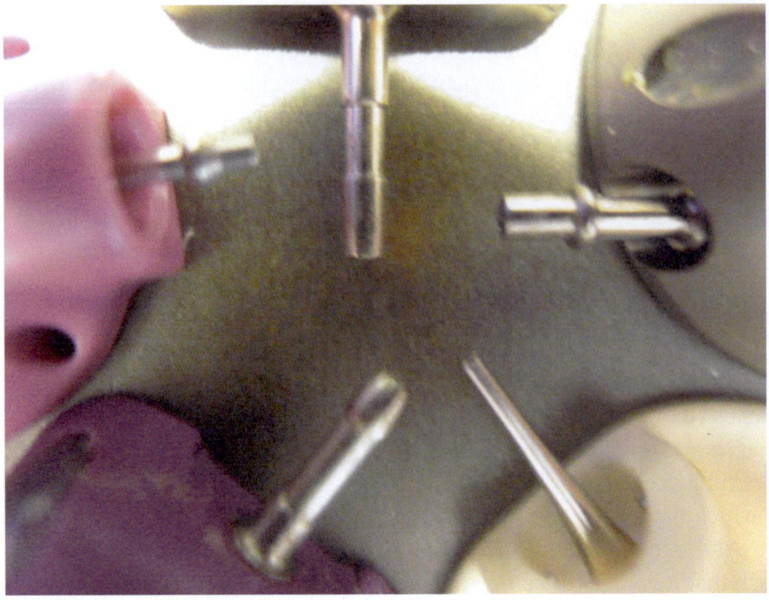

Fig. 3.23 Various shapes of support cannulas

but in practice does not work, since the path of the needle tip is not determined by the user's puncture direction, but by the geometry of the bevel. Accordingly, the first bent segment of the needle does not move in the direction of puncture, but at an angle to it. Thus, the Huber bevel planes just like a standard bevel (Fig. 3.14). The improved Huber needles available today are better because certain areas of the bevel have been blunted, reducing the tendency to plane, as there is no longer a sharp edge. The bend in the needle shaft above the bevel is functionally superfluous.

Also in 1988, a novel port needle was first reported that is virtually non-coring up to needle size 20G (Haindl et al. 1995) (Fig. 3.24). The fact that even with virtually non-coring needles, particle formation occasionally occurs is due to the manufacturing process: needles are made from welded tubes, and the weld seam creates a small section of the circumference with greater hardness than the rest. Regardless of the method used to blunt the edge of the rear bevel eye, there will always be a difference in performance between the softer and harder sections of the needle tube. Therefore, a needle should never be judged based on a single sample.

Attempts with pencil-point needles were largely unsuccessful. While the use of pencil-point needles can completely prevent coring and particle formation, the puncture is painful for the patient and acceptance is low. To address this, pencil-point needles with an additional three-facet bevel at the tip were developed, which solve this problem. However, their production is very complex.

The development of non-coring needles took place at a time when the majority of port catheters were made of plastic, and the inner surface of the port was also plastic. As attention increasingly focused on particle formation, most

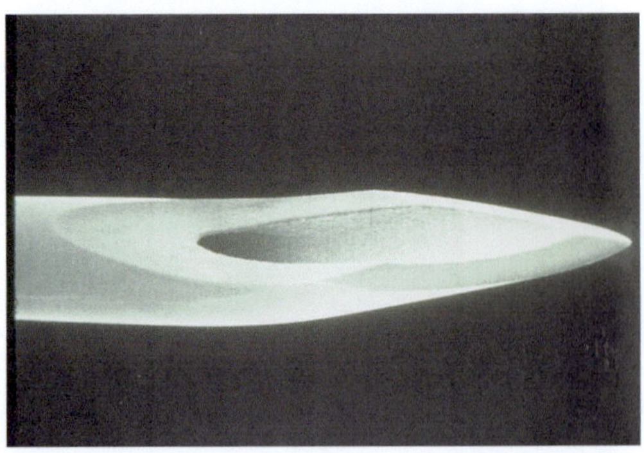

Fig. 3.24 Non-coring needle (Surecan, Braun)

manufacturers began to integrate particle-resistant, i.e., hard, bases or chambers into their ports, usually made of titanium and, in some cases, ceramic. This solved the problem of particle release from the port housing, but introduced a new issue.

Non-coring needles generally have a relatively long bevel, meaning the tip is relatively thin. As a result, if the needle strikes the base with some force, a hook can form at the tip (Fig. 3.23). When the needle is withdrawn, this hook can damage the port membrane, potentially negating the longevity advantage of the non-coring bevel.

A solution to this problem has been developed (Fig. 3.26). The deformations of the tip shown in Figs. 3.25 and 3.27 were produced using a testing machine applying identical forces and speeds. The needle that does not bend is also non-coring, though at the stage of development shown, it still requires slightly more insertion force. The development has been described and published, but has not attracted interest from port manufacturers.

Port needles are also potentially infectious after use, so, as with other needles, user protection against injury is required by accident prevention regulation TRBA 250 and EU Directive 2000/54/EC. Manufacturers offer various solutions to this requirement (Figs. 3.28 and 3.29).

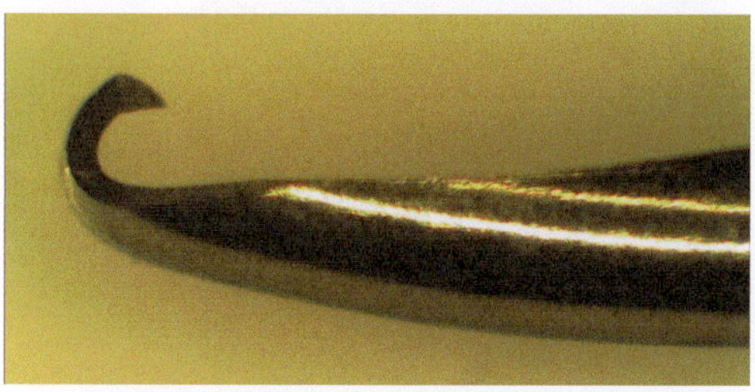

Fig. 3.25 Hook formation after striking a hard port base

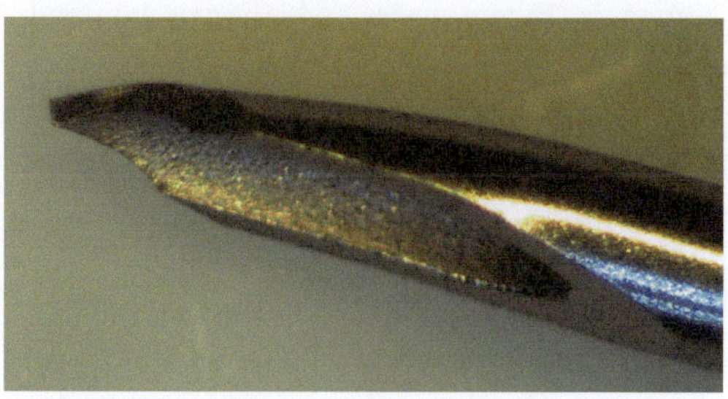

Fig. 3.26 Hook-resistant needle bevel

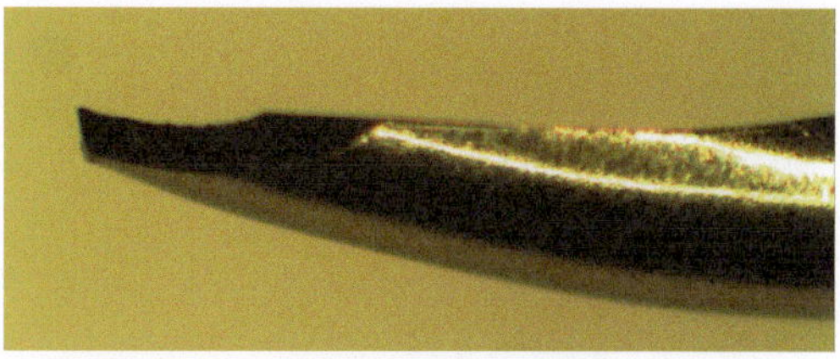

Fig. 3.27 Same after striking a hard port base (same force as in Fig. 3.25)

3.4.7 Introducer Systems

While catheter placement via cutdown of the cephalic vein does not require additional instruments, all other access routes require an introducer system. Systems using the Seldinger technique have become established, in which a relatively thin needle is first used to puncture the blood vessel, and then, after insertion of a Seldinger wire, the needle is removed to prevent vascular injury. The catheter is rarely introduced directly over the Seldinger wire, as dilation of the catheter tract and the use of a usually splitable sheath are generally required. The sheath is essential, especially for silicone catheters, as these cannot be advanced through tissue (Fig. 3.30).

Recently, introducer systems with valves have also been introduced (Fig. 3.31) to prevent air embolism. Since port catheter implantation is always an elective procedure, it should not be a problem to prevent air embolism by ensuring positive central venous pressure. In any case, introducer sheaths with valves are advantageous in that the procedure becomes less bloody. The valves are split and removed along with the sheath.

3.5 Outlook

The preceding discussion can only cover a relatively small number of recent developments in the field of port catheters. Many initiatives, such

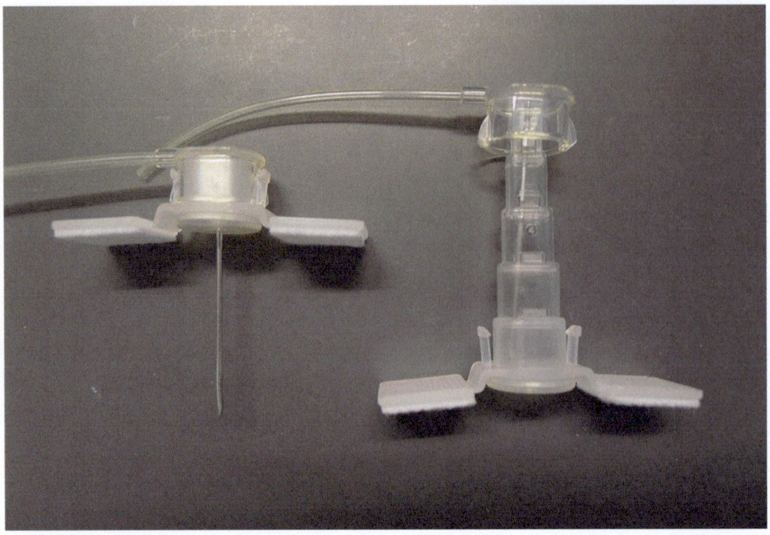

Fig. 3.28 Fresenius safety needle

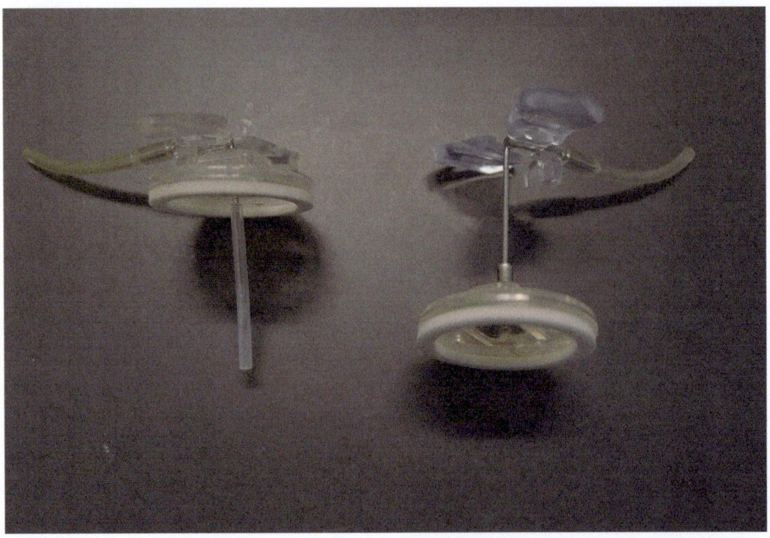

Fig. 3.29 Braun safety needle

as electronic locating devices for port catheters, have never reached market maturity because their benefits are clearly insufficient and the associated problems, for example in MRI, cannot be easily resolved. Other innovations, such as an embolism-proof catheter, remain unavailable despite some promising initial attempts. It should also be noted that the pace of innovation in the port catheter market has noticeably slowed in recent years, which can be readily explained by falling prices.

The listing of problems is intended to improve port catheters, but should by no means give the impression that these are products with unacceptably high risks. Nevertheless, it must be pointed out that those who implant port catheters are often not confronted with their complications. This has led to an unfortunate trend

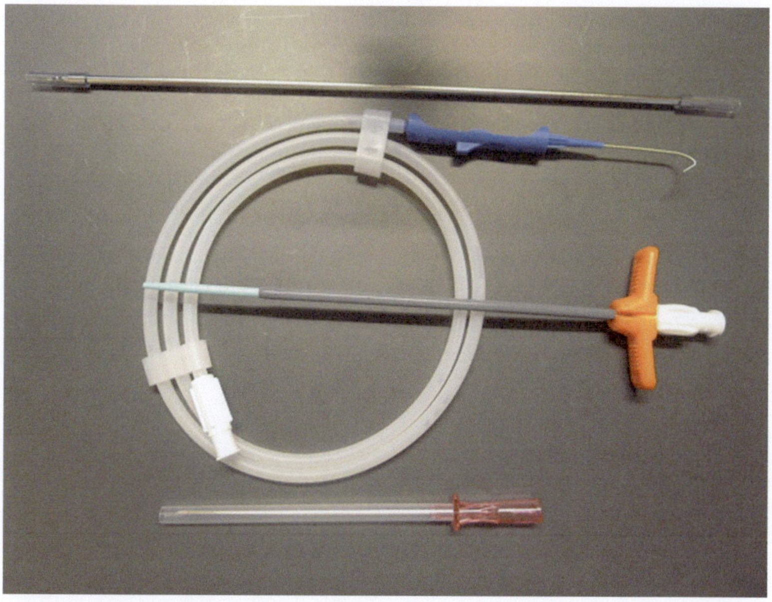

Fig. 3.30 Introducer set with splitable sheath

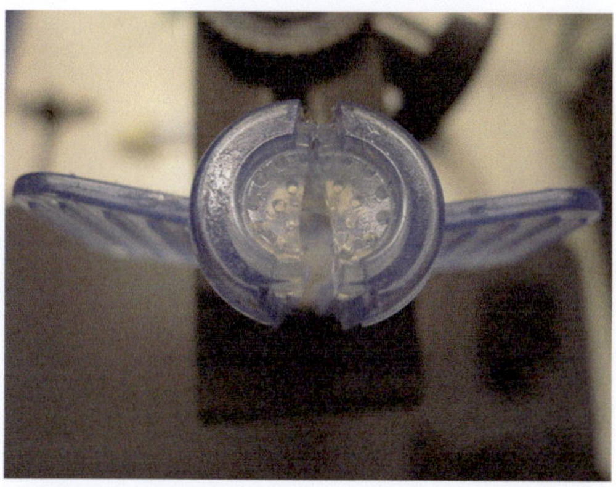

Fig. 3.31 Split sheath valve

toward selecting the least expensive port catheter system. Therefore, it is incumbent upon users to remain vigilant and to continually compare the complication rates of different port systems.

References

Blackshear PJ, Dorman FD, Blackshear PL, Varco RL, Buchwald HA (1970) permanently implantable self-recycling low flow constant rate multipurpose infusion pump of simple design. Surgical forum 21:136–137

Ecoff L, Barone RM, Simons RM (1983) Implantable infusion port (Port-A-Cath). NITA. Nov–Dec;6(6):406–8

Haindl H (1989) Technical Complications of Port Catheter Systems Reg Cancer Treat 2:238–242

Haindl H, Schmoll E, Willmann G (1995) Ein neues Portkathetersystem aus Aluminiumoxidkeramik. Biomedizinische Technik. Biomedical Engineering 40(3):42–49

Haindl H, Müller H (1988) Eine atraumatische Nadel für die Punktion von Ports und Pumpen. Klinische Wochenschrift 66(20):1006–1009

Haeder L, Jähne J (2013) Indikation, Technik und Komplikationen der Portimplantation Chirurg. 84:572–579 https://doi.org/10.1007/s00104-012-2408-5. © Springer-Verlag Berlin Heidelberg

Janßen R (1989) Vergleichende Untersuchung von Portsystemen. Dissertation, Universität Münster

Kurul S, Saip P, Aydin T (2002) Totally implantable venous-access ports: local problems and extravasation injury. The Lancet Oncology 3(11):684–692

Patel GS, Jain K, Kumar R, Strickland AH, Pellegrini L, Slavotinek J, Eaton M, McLeay W, Price T, Ly M, Ullah S, Koczwara B, Kichenadasse G, Karapetis CS (2014) Comparison of peripherally inserted central venous catheters (PICC) versus subcutaneously implanted port-chamber catheters by complication and cost for patients receiving chemotherapy for non-haematological malignancies. Supportive care in cancer: official journal of the Multinational Association of Supportive Care in Cancer 22(1):121–128

Müller H, Zierski J (1988) Die Huber-Nadel als Spezialkanüle für die Punktion von implantierten

Ports und Pumpen--ein Irrtum in zahlreichen Variationen. Klinische Wochenschrift 66(19):963–969

Niederhuber JE, Ensminger W, Gyves JW, Liepman M, Doan K, Cozzi E (1982) Totally implanted venous and arterial access system to replace external catheters in cancer treatment. Surgery 92(4):706–712

Ng F, Mastoroudes H, Paul E, Davies N, Tibballs J, Hochhauser D, Mayer A, Begent R, Meyer TA (2007) comparison of Hickman line- and Port-a-Cath-associated complications in patients with solid tumours undergoing chemotherapy. Clinical oncology (Royal College of Radiologists (Great Britain)) 19(7):551–556

Sharp Nicole E, Knott EM, Thomas P, Rivard DC, St Peter, SD (2014) Burden of complications from needle penetration of plastic ports in children. Journal of pediatric surgery 49(5):763–765

Pollmann D, Schildhauer S, Lüftner D (2002–2021) 14 Venenzugänge, Kathetersysteme (Ports): Portsystem. © ONKODIN 2002–2021 | ISSN: 2193-6021

Teichgräber KU, Pfitzmann R, Hofmann, HAF (2014). Portsysteme als integraler Bestandteil von Chemotherapien Ärzteblatt 01/2014

4 Indication and Preparation of the Patient for Port Implantation and Explantation

Roland Hennes

Determining the indication is one of the most demanding tasks for any surgeon. Timing, surgical intervention, the surgeon's qualifications for the procedure, anesthesia technique, and other aspects all factor into the decision-making process. In addition, a standardized and well-considered preparation of the patient, including all necessary and extended diagnostic measures, is the next crucial step for the success of the surgical procedure.

4.1 Indications for Placement of a Port Catheter

Determining the indication for a surgical procedure is among the most critical responsibilities of the consulting physician. The indication for placement of a port catheter primarily concerns patients with oncological diseases, but also applies to patients with intestinal disorders, immunodeficiencies, metabolic diseases, or conditions that require long-term medication administration, such as in pain therapy. The indication may also be as simple as difficulty obtaining blood samples in patients with poor venous status, For these patients, a port provides a reliable means to ensure regular blood sampling. Although, in general, blood sampling via the port are dicouraged in patients with otherwise good veins to prevent compromising the system (e.g., occlusion). When difficulty in obtaining blood samples is the indication for port placement, competent port care is essential. After each blood sampling, the the port should be thoroughly flushed using the push-and-go technique with saline solution. We recommend at least 20 ml of saline.

Another indication that has become standard in modern diagnostics for oncology patients is the administration of contrast agents via the port catheter during CT or MRI examinations. Especially in patients with very poor venous access—as described above—the ability to administer contrast agents via the port catheter offers substantial benefits by avoiding unnecessary forearm punctures. However, for contrast administration via a port catheter, it is necessary to implant a high-pressure system that is specifically approved for this purpose. In this regard, it is worth critically considering whether high-pressure ports should be established as standard in oncology patients if they are not already in use. At the Heidelberg Port Center, high-pressure ports have been exclusively implanted as standard for the past 12 years to ensure this function for patients. Of course, the

R. Hennes (✉)
Klinik für Allgemein-, Viszeral- und Transplantationschirurgie, Universitätsklinikum Heidelberg, Heidelberg, Germany
e-mail: Roland.Hennes@med.uni-heidelberg.de

R. Hennes (ed.), *Port Surgery*, https://doi.org/10.1007/978-3-662-70624-4_4

price differences between high-pressure and non-high-pressure ports must be weighed. In our opinion, however, the quality of patient care should take precedence, and the price differences are not so significant as to justify withholding the option of contrast administration via a port catheter from patients.

The indications mentioned above for adults also apply to children, where similar clinical pictures are generally observed. In children, additional indications include regular substitution therapies such as antibiotics and nutritional solutions, for example in cystic fibrosis or other genetic disorders. The port is also used, for instance, during prolonged radiation therapy for sedation and anesthesia in young children. If a port catheter is not tolerated, placement of a Hickman catheter is a good alternative for children (Hennes and Hofman 2016).

Indications for Placement of a Port Catheter

- Chemotherapy
- Parenteral nutrition
- Regular administration of medications and nutritional solutions
- Administration of contrast agents for CT and MRI diagnostics
- Blood sampling in cases of severely compromised venous access
- Administration of blood products and other infusion solutions
- Blood collection in patients with very poor venous access

Naturally, the indication must be discussed in detail with the patient. In particular, it is important for oncology patients, especially those from gynecological backgrounds, to be well informed that the indication for a port catheter is not solely for chemotherapy, but also—as outlined above—for diagnostic purposes or blood sampling. In our practice, the duration of port catheter placement for conditions such as breast cancer is at least 1–2 years, until it can be reliably confirmed that the port is no longer needed (Hennes and Hofmann 2016).

It is essential to ensure that patients fully understand the indication so that they can develop a positive attitude toward the port catheter.

4.2 Preparation of the Patient

The establishment of an indication is accompanied by the responsible preparation of the patient. Based on the course of therapy and medical history, the appropriate timing must be determined in consultation with the patient, the treating colleagues, and the implanting clinic or practice. It is advisable to standardize the preparatory measures and to inform all parties involved accordingly.

Checklist for Patient Preparation for Port Implantation

- **Patient data**:
  - First and last name
  - Date of birth
  - Telephone number
- **Surgical data:**
  - Diagnoses
  - Planned procedure (port, port explantation, Hickman [single-lumen, double-lumen], Demers, double-chamber port)
  - Planned side and site
  - Planned anesthesia (patients scheduled for placement of a port catheter or Hickman catheter can generally undergo the procedure under local anesthesia and **DO NOT** need to be fasting)
- **Medically and nursing-relevant patient information:**
  - Infectious diseases (MRSA, VRE, etc.)
  - Parameters requiring monitoring

- Conditions relevant to positioning, such as hemiplegia, paraplegia, and existing fractures, especially of the spine
- Special drains
- Tracheostomy tube
- Impaired compliance due to psychiatric, psychosomatic disorders, or dementia
- Procedure-specific documents and diagnostics
- Timely organization and notification regarding required blood products for the surgical procedure
- Required findings, informed consent for the surgical procedure such as anesthesia, and, if applicable, ultrasound findings or advanced imaging (CT, MRI)
- Medication use, especially anticoagulants (timely discontinuation)
- Transport management

For all central venous catheters, it must be ensured that venous drainage to the heart via the subclavian vein, jugular vein, and, if applicable, via the femoral vein to the inferior vena cava is unobstructed. In cases of thrombosis, previous surgeries, or radiation in the thoracic or inguinal region, diagnostic evaluation with ultrasound or advanced imaging should be performed beforehand. The choice of the operative side must be made carefully after assessing all findings (Biffi et al. 2009). This decision affects the surgical outcome and the intraoperative course. Current infection parameters must also be considered. The surgical site should show no signs of infection.

From the perspective of anesthesia and surgery, coagulation values are important for preparation, as are all other parameters required for anesthesia (see Chap. 8). All information such as comorbidities should be highlighted, and in particular, infections or colonization with multidrug-resistant organisms must be verified and clarified in detail with the surgical team and the operating clinic (practice) for surgical planning.

Especially for outpatient surgery or procedures under local anesthesia, the patient must be thoroughly informed about the process on the day of surgery. At the Port Center of the Department of Surgery, University Hospital, patients are given a port brochure during the consent process, which provides all contact information and details relevant to the day of surgery. We repeatedly observe that patients whose indication and consent were obtained externally and who are to undergo surgery explicitly under local anesthesia are instructed to remain fasting on the day of surgery. For patients, not having breakfast is often a significant burden, as it can affect their circulation and blood glucose levels.

In accordance with the checklist, all comorbidities and allergies should, of course, be clarified prior to surgery to ensure patient safety. For patients undergoing surgery under analgosedation or general anesthesia, it is necessary—according to the requirements for outpatient surgery under § 105—that the patient is accompanied on the way home after the procedure and is not left alone at home, but is supervised by a relative or adult. Therefore, travel arrangements, return transport, and patient accompaniment are also important aspects to ensure the safe care of port patients.

As part of patient preparation, it is, of course, essential to have the appropriate port catheter materials available. While some hospitals use a "standard port" for all patients—which we do not recommend at the Port Center—since different body constitutions require different port chamber sizes, we keep four different port chamber sizes and various port catheters available at the Port Center Heidelberg. The different port chamber sizes allow the port to be adapted to the individual patient's constitution. For example, a female patient weighing 39 kg with short bowel syndrome may be at risk of a transmural ulcer if a larger port is used and the skin over the port is very tight. For such patients, we have a small port that avoids this problem. Conversely, in a patient weighing 200 kg, a small port—especially if not implanted close to the skin surface—may be very difficult to access, necessitating repeated punctures and thereby increasing the risk of infection. Therefore, it is important to select the port chamber size so that port access is as easy and stress-free for the patient as possible.

For optimal surgical performance, it is first necessary to determine, through patient examination, the best site for implantation of the port catheter and port chamber. Previous surgeries on the shoulder, thoracic procedures, or prior operations or thromboses in the access area for port catheter placement—such as the subclavian vein, jugular vein, or femoral vein—require clear preoperative evaluation by ultrasound to rule out thrombosis. In cases of difficult venous conditions, angiographic CT may also be necessary. Skin changes, such as inflammation or infection at the intended implantation site, also preclude port placement at that location.

4.3 Documentation, Consent, and Information for Patients and Relatives

In addition to obtaining consent with signatures from the patient or their legal representative and the physician providing the information, this document must be carefully kept together with all other patient records. At the Port Center Heidelberg, we consider it essential to inform patients and their relatives about all aspects of the surgical procedure in advance through our port brochure and comprehensive counseling. The aim is also to provide patients with a sense of security so that they can approach the procedure with confidence. Informing relatives is equally important. (Fig. 4.1).

4.4 Indications for Port Explantation

Careful assessment of the indication for port explantation is always essential. There are various indications for port explantation, most commonly in the context of a port infection or at the end of therapy. In addition, explantation is indicated in cases of non-functioning port catheters. Not least, patient preference plays a role when patients request removal of the port (Fischer et al. 2008). As previously mentioned, the port catheter is also used for CT or MRI diagnostics with contrast administration. Therefore, we recommend not removing the port catheter immediately after completion of chemotherapy. Unfortunately, we often see recurrences, necessitating a repeat procedure to implant a new port catheter. This is not always a straightforward task, as previous surgeries may have caused scarring, for example, if the cephalic vein has already been used and is no longer available (see Chap. 16).

For this reason, the indication for port explantation should be determined very carefully in consultation with the patient and the treating physicians. Port explantation is not always a "beginner's procedure," but must be carefully planned and performed with a sound surgical strategy. Especially with long-term indwelling ports, adhesions are frequently encountered, which can lead to catheter rupture. This, in turn, usually necessitates interventional measures, requiring the radiologist to remove the remaining port catheter in a second procedure.

Tears of the brachiocephalic vein are also possible (see Chap. 16). Port explantation in cases of long-term indwelling ports (>5 years) should be performed by an experienced surgeon.

For long-term indwelling port catheters, phlebography can be helpful in assessing the extent of adhesions. Preparation for port explantation follows the same principles as for port implantation, with attention to patient counseling, correct indication, laboratory diagnostics, and other items as outlined in the checklist. In general, we recommend port explantation after a maximum of five years. If there is still an indication for a port after five years, a port catheter exchange can be performed. As described by Dr. Haindl (Hennes and Hofman 2016), material fatigue occurs after five years, such as pitting corrosion at the port catheter coupling between the port chamber and the port catheter, or other degenerative changes in the material.

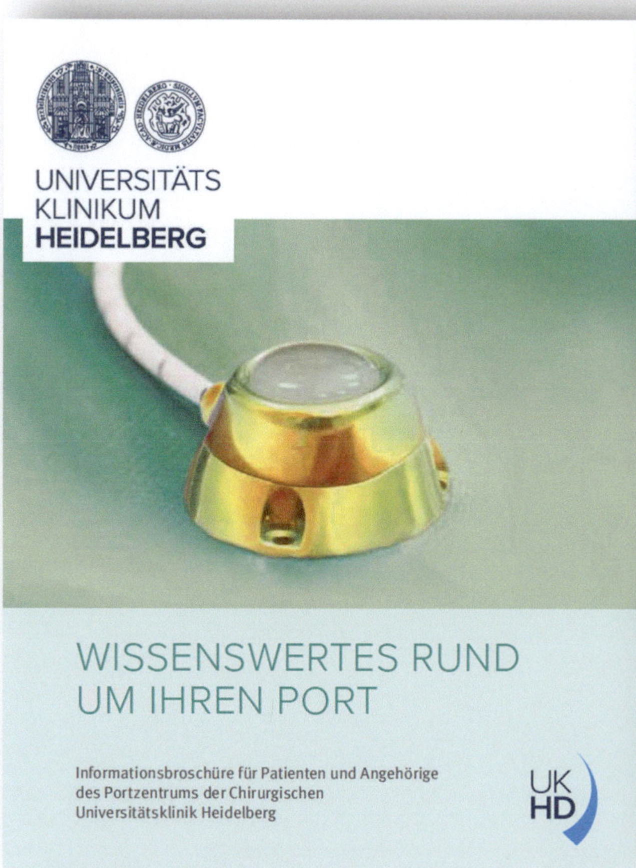

Fig. 4.1 Port brochure for informing the patient and their relatives

References

Biffi R, Orsi F, Pozzi S et al (2009) Best choice of central venous insertion site for the prevention of catheter-related complications in adult patients who need cancer therapy: a randomized trial. Ann Oncol 20:935–940

Fischer L, Knebel P, Schroder S et al (2008) Reasons for explantation of totally implantable access ports: a multivariate analysis of 385 consecutive patients. Ann Surg Oncol 15:1124–1129

Hennes R, Hofmann H (2016) Ports. Springer. ISBN 978-3-662-43640-0

Organization of the Surgical Process for Optimization of Patient Care

5

Felix Johannes Jost

▶ **Trailer** Organizing a surgical procedure is often challenging for all involved and thus represents a daily test of personal skills and resilience. This burden can be reduced by applying systematic standards. For smooth execution and optimal surgical outcomes, the collaboration of a well-trained surgical team is absolutely essential. Every team member should be aware of their role and contribute to process optimization and workflow to the best of their knowledge and ability. This is the only way to ensure high-quality patient care, especially when local anesthesia is used, as patients are aware of all staff actions and any uncertainty or unprofessional communication can lead to anxiety.

5.1 Introduction

Procedures ensuring patient saftey are commonly well known and documented; however, some important processes are often neglected, especially in shorter interventions such as port catheter implantation or Hickman catheter placement. Nevertheless, they are essential both legally and for patient safety.

F. J. Jost (✉)
Universitätsklinikum Heidelberg, Heidelberg, Germany
e-mail: felixjohannes.jost@med.uni-heidelberg.de

Mandatory measures include thorough patient education regarding procedural specifications, a team time-out or a comparable preoperative checklist, and adequate postoperative care, particularly in an ambulant setting. Ideally, the patient, their relatives, the treating department, as well as the responsible nursing service are provided with information and documentation materials regardingthe implanted product. Since trained handling, especially of port systems, is not always guaranteed. Thus comprehensive education is required, as improper handling poses a significant risk to the patient. Patient safety must always be the top priority.

Both patients and staff benefit from well-practiced preparation, respectful interaction, gentle and expert execution, and optimized postoperative care. Interdisciplinary collaboration must be emphasized, as it ensures the quality of patient care.

The following section outlines an organizational plan with all necessary measures.

5.2 Procedural Planning

A structured and organized planning of any surgical procedure is crucial for its smooth execution, patient safety, and patient satisfaction.

Firstly, this necessitates a thorough and complete surgical consultation, including the evaluation of all required preoperative investigations

R. Hennes (ed.), *Port Surgery*, https://doi.org/10.1007/978-3-662-70624-4_5

(vascular CT or vascular ultrasound, blood tests to determine surgery-relevant laboratory values, such ascoagulation and infection parameters).

For women of childbearing age, it is essential to inquire about possible pregnancy. In case of uncertainty a pregnency test should be performed to adhere to general guidelines of radiation protection.

Choice of Anesthesia Method

One of the key questions for the patient is the choice of anesthesia for the surgical procedure. Available options include local anesthesia, analgosedation in combination with local anesthesia, or general anesthesia (see Chap. 8 Anesthesia for Port Procedures).

Important decision factors, in addition to the patient's general and health status, include psychological factors and the patient's preferences. For many patients without a medical background, undergoing surgery while conscious is a significant challenge and burden. Here, objective and empathetic counseling is essential.

Furthermore, careful inspection of the surgical site is essential. Previous surgeries in the area of the infraclavicular fossa, shoulder, or clavicle can complicate or even preclude the procedure. Absolute contraindications include, the presence of thrombosis in the subclavian vein or a dialysis shunt in the arm on the side to be operated. In such cases, the contralateral side or, if necessary, the groin should be preferred for the procedure. In the presence of breast cancer, the affected side should be avoided to prevent further impairment of lymphatic drainage.

Outpatient treatment is only possible if the patient is in a safe and supportive social environment. If this is not the case, inpatient treatment is required.

5.3 Organization on the Day of Surgery

Ideally, the patient should not arrive fasting on the day of the planned procedure under local anesthesia. Lying in a supine position during the operation and possible underlying conditions pose a significant risk of complications and can negatively affect the patient's well-being if fasting.

In an outpatient setting, patient preparation is best carried out in a day clinic or equivalent facility. Such an institution can admit the patient in advance an perform all necessary preoperative preparations, including compilation of patient-specific documents. In addition, the day clinic can provide the patient with procedural details and assist with changing clothes and shaving the surgical site.

Short communication pathways between the surgical department and the day clinic facilitate quick and flexible adjustments to the surgical schedule, which is often necessary in hospitals performing numerous short procedures across multiple operating rooms.

It is advisable to schedule patients who require isolation due to resistant pathogens (MRSA, MRGN, Clostridia, etc.) at the end of the surgical program.

For highly infectious agents, such as SARS-CoV-2 or norovirus, it must be determined whether port placement is urgently indicated or if the procedure can be deferred.

5.4 Preoperative Checklists

Preoperative checklists (Fig. 5.1), such as a team time-out, are among the most important comprehensive safety measures performed by the entire surgical team.

Using a preoperative checklist, the responsible nurse can verify the completeness of all required patient documents before entering the operating room. This includes signed surgical and, if applicable, anesthesiology consent forms, current laboratory results with relevant previous findings, as well as completed imaging studies.

When performing general anesthesia, such as intubation anesthesia, laryngeal mask ventilation, or analgosedation, it is essential to confirm that the patient is fully fasted.

Verifying the patient's name, date of birth, the type and location of the planned surgery helps prevent identification errors. In

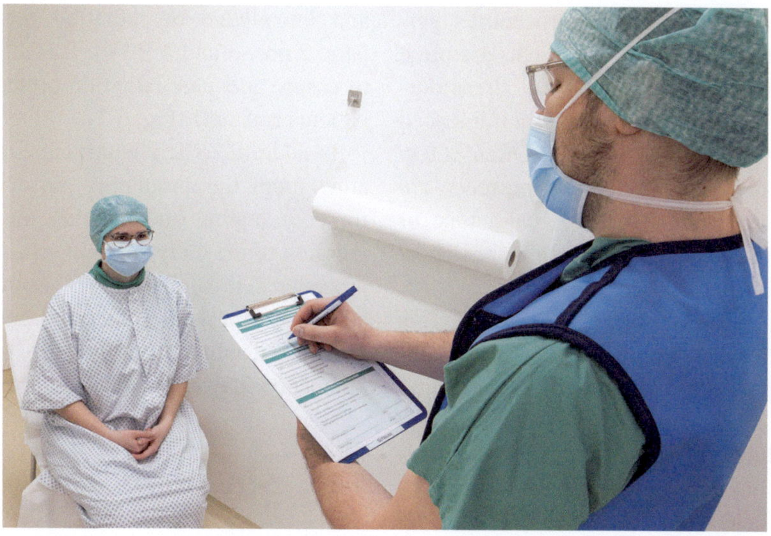

Fig. 5.1 Time-out and documentation on the time-out form

addition, it is essential to review any allergies, intolerances, infectious pre-existing conditions, and presence of implants such as joint endoprostheses, pacemakers, or defibrillators. In allows for the timely recognition and prevention of, potential problems before entering the operating area. Proper and thorough preoperative checks make a significant contribution to patient safety and significantly reduce the incidence of errors and complications (Á. Oszvald et al. 2012).

A team time-out before the start of surgical measures is essential and must be carried out and documented consistently without any exceptions. All staff present in the operating room participate in this process. Thus all tasks should be interrupted to concentrate fully on the team member leading the process.

First, members of the surgical team introduce themselves including name and function. If all participants are acquainted and no new or unfamiliar staff present, a simple confirmation is sufficient. Secondly, the patient's identity and the planned procedure must be clearly stated. This includes the type of surgical intervention, as well as the precise location and side. If any special circumstances or critical situations are anticipated, they should be detailed as well. Once all remaining questions have been clarified, the team time-out is considered complete. For legally compliantdocumentation, the process should ideally be recorded on a standardized form and signed by the surgeon, anesthesiologist, and operating room nurse. Studies have shown that conducting a team time-out not only significantly reduces treatment errors (Fudickar et al. 2012; Haugen et al. 2013), but also sharpens the staff's focus on comprehensive, responsible, and risk-aware patient care (Birgit Weingessel et al. 2017), with minimal time and personnel effort.

Especially for port catheter placement, it is important not only to verify the intended side but, in selected cases, also consider placement in the groin. Careful inquiry about previous surgeries and thorough preoperative evaluation of the planned insertion site can help avoid many complications In some cases, preoperative angiological evaluation is necessary. This may involve ruling out thrombosis by ultrasound or angio-CT, as well as general assessment of venous return and potential collateral circulation.

5.5 Circulating Nurse Duties

During surgery, a well-trained operating room team is crucial in many respects. Careful execution of circulating nurse responsibilities is crucial for the success of procedures performed under local anesthesia. Patients are often exposed to significant psychological stress during surgery. This can be substantially influenced and alleviated by the nursing staff. Often, a few reassuring words and an attentive presence are enough to help patients relax. A calm tone of voice and empathetic communication are important in this context. In addition to patient care, the nurse is responsible for documentation. This includes the legally required surgical documentation as well as procedure-specific documentation for port placement. The operative report is the responsibility of the surgeon. A standardized "port summary" is helpful in this regard (Fig. 5.2). In addition to patient data, this form records implantation details including size, manufacturer, and lot number. This information is provided on stickers accompanying all standard port systems, facilitating direct documentation. The accessed vein and surgical technique should also be recorded. The well-established practice of intraoperative chest fluoroscopy to determine and verify catheter placement is a delegable task underradiation protection regulations(§ 24 para. 2 RöV). It may therefore be performed by the circulating nurse under physician supervision, provided the nurse has the necessary qualifications (§ 24 para. 2 no. 1 or no. 2 RöV) and knowledge of radiation protection (§ 24 para. 2 nos. 3 and 4 RöV). It is always essential to ensure adequate radiation protection for both patients and staff (Fig. 5.3).

In addition to active participation in the operating room, the circulating nurse is responsible for coordinating and ensuring the smooth progression of the daily surgical schedule. For short procedures, it is important to ensure timely preparation of the next patient and communication-with the cleaning staff. Here, too, the advantages of a nearby day clinic located become evident.

5.6 Scrub Nurse Duties

Despite the short duration of the procedure and the relatively small set of instruments, the role of the scrub nurse can be demanding. Many surgical steps must be anticipated and often demand a precise and delicate technique. Depending on the size and condition of the vein, microsurgical techniques such as the use of guidewires can pose significant challenges, especially for less experienced staff. Certain procedural steps can be executed efficiently only through close cooperation between the surgeon and the scrub nurse. In addition to confident and anticipatory instrument handling, precise

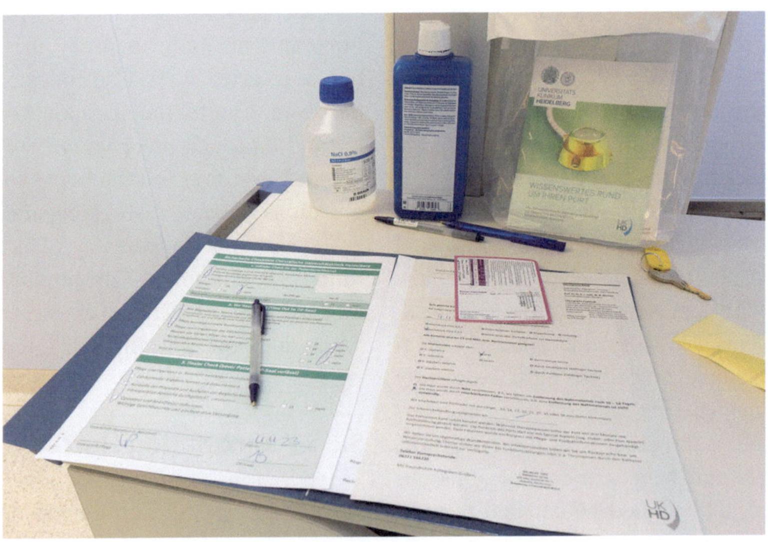

Fig. 5.2 Documentation and information for patient and relatives

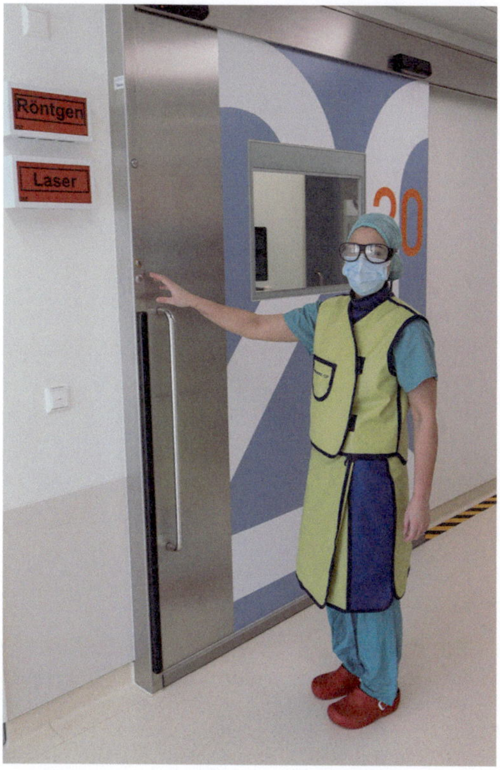

Fig. 5.3 Personal protective equipment for radiation protection as recommended by the Radiation Protection Ordinance

assistance during catheter insertion—whether using the modified Seldinger technique, the conventional Seldinger technique, or by venous cutdown—is crucial. Delays in instrument handling can negatively impact the surgical workflow.

5.7 Postoperative Patient Care

Postoperative care of the patient is highly dependent on the type of anesthesia used. An outpatient managed under local anesthesia with a stable social environment can leave the clinic just a few minutes after surgery after discharged by the surgeon. It is essential to provide the patient with comprehensive information. This includes instructions for home and primary care follow-up, as well as fundamental rules for handling the newly implanted port catheter. Benefits and risks arising from poor hygiene during port access should be made unequivocally clear. The medical staff is responsible for the use of the port and adherence to hygiene standards; however, the patient should also be encouraged to monitor the correct use of their port. Providing the manufacturer's implant card and a fully completed port record (see Fig. 5.2) facilitates effective collaboration with outpatient and hospital-based oncologists. In addition to complete patient data, it is important to include the recommended needle length, the manufacturer's model designation, and the batch number. For a Hickman catheter, documentation of the number of lumens along with the batch and reference numbers is essential. Patients are advised to bring these documents to every medical appointment.

For most patients, surgery is an exceptional situation. It is therefore understandable that they may not remember all the information provided to them. Therefore our clinic has developed an information sheet answering the most frequently asked questions briefly and concisely.

To ensure optimal information transfer to patients, we have created a port brochure at the Port Center of the Department of Surgery at Heidelberg University Hospital, specifically tailored to address patients' questions and concerns. This brochure is regularly updated to reflect the latest standards (see Fig. 5.4). Many fundamental questions are answered here in a clear and comprehensive manner.

If general anesthesia has been administered, postoperative monitoring is absolutely necessary. Even before surgery, for outpatient procedures under general anesthesia, it must be ensured that home monitoring is possible. After observation in the recovery room or day clinic, the patient should not be left unattended for the next 24 h. If this cannot be guaranteed, inpatient admission must be arranged prior to surgery. During postoperative monitoring, noninvasive blood pressure measurement, ECG, and oxygen saturation monitoring are required. The patient may only leave the clinic after oral intake of food and fluids, spontaneous urination, and discharge by both the surgeon and an anesthesiologist.

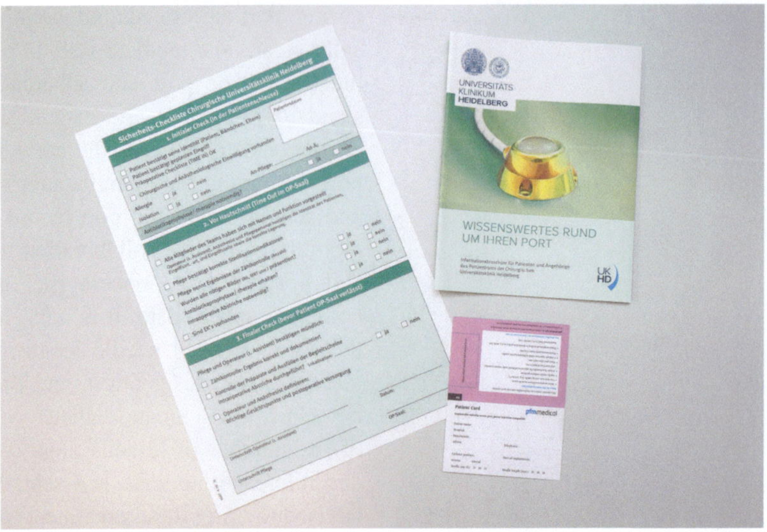

Fig. 5.4 Time-out checklist, port brochure, and port card

In general, patients should refrain from sports activities for the first 10 days after surgery. Similarly, physical work, especially overhead activities and heavy lifting, should be avoided. As the skin is routinely closed with a "buried" continuous intradermal suture, showering is permitted 48 h after surgery. After showering, a fresh, dry dressing should simply be applied. Bathing and swimming should be avoided until the wound has completely healed.

If a port needle remains in place, special caution is required due to the potential entry point for pathogens and the increased risk of injury from the needle. In this case, even showering with a waterproof dressing is only recommended to a limited extent.

References

Appelhoff B, Moser L (2020) Intraoperative und Postoperative Betreuung von Portpatienten. In: Hennes R (ed) Portpflege, 1st edn. Springer, Berlin, pp 61–66

Fantl B (2020) Wundversorgung und Verbandswechsel. In: Hennes R (ed) Portpflege, 1st edn. Springer, Berlin, pp 51–60

Fudickar A, Hörle K, Wiltfang J, Bein B (2012) The effect of the WHO surgical safety checklist on complication rate and communication. 109(42):695–701

Haugen AS, Murugesh S, Haaverstad R et al (2013) A survey of surgical team members' perceptions of near misses and attitudes towards Time Out protocols. BMC Surg 13:46

Hennes R, Hofmann F (2016) Ports. Springer Hennes and Hofmann 2016, Appelhoff and Moser 2020, Fantl 2020 are not cited in the text. Please provide the citations. All these references readet as further readings

Oszvald A, Vatter H, Byhahn C, Seifert V, Güresir E (2012) "Team time-out" and surgical safety—experiences in 12,390 neurosurgical patients. Departments of Neurosurgery and Anesthesiology, Intensive Care Medicine, and Pain Therapy, Johann Wolfgang Goethe University

Weingessel B, Haas M, Vécsei C (2017) Pia Veronika Vécsei-Marlovits Clinical risk management—a 3-year experience of team timeout in 18 081 ophthalmic patients. https://doi.org/10.1111/aos.13155

Part II

Performing Port Procedures

6 Procedure-Specific Access Anatomy for Port Procedures

Roland Hennes

▶ The implantation of central venous catheters, including port systems, requires both comprehensive and region-specific anatomical knowledge to ensure proper surgical planning and execution. This chapter outlines the three principal anatomical regions commonly used for port catheter implantation.

The surgical access routes for central venous catheter implantation are conventionally classified into three distinct anatomical regions:

1. Fossa clavi-deltoideo-pectoralis (= Mohrenheim's fossa)
2. Lateral cervical region, with visualization of the neurovascular structures in the lateral neck area
3. Inguinal region, with the superficial and deep neurovascular structures below the inguinal ligament

Within these three anatomical regions, almost all central venous catheters can be placed. For information detailing the anatomy and access routes of interventional port placement in the lumbar and hepatic veins, please refer to Chap. 15.

R. Hennes (✉)
Klinik für Allgemein-, Viszeral- und Transplantationschirurgie, Universitätsklinikum Heidelberg, Heidelberg, Germany
e-mail: Roland.Hennes@med.uni-heidelberg.de

1) Mohrenheim's fossa (Fossa clavi-deltoideo-pectoralis)

The anatomically simplest and safest access for placement of a central venous catheter into the cephalic vein is via Mohrenheim's fossa (Fig. 6.1).

Mohrenheim's fossa is bordered by the deltoid muscle, the pectoralis major muscle, and the clavicle. The cephalic vein runs cranially within the deltoideopectoral groove and, after passing through the clavipectoral fascia, drains into the subclavian vein at the level of Mohrenheim's fossa. The incision site for the procedure should be selected based on well-defined anatomical landmarks. These include the clavicle, the medial margin of the humeral head, and the palpable fossa clavi-deltoideo-pectoralis. Placing the index finger on these landmarks provides orientation cranially, toward the external jugular vein.

This approach provides the quickest access to the cephalic vein, which is typically found in Mohrenheim's fossa after dissecting the fatty fascia above it (Fig. 6.2).

As with all venous pathways, considerable anatomical variation can be observed in the region of Mohrenheim's fossa. If the cephalic vein cannot be found centrally in Mohrenheim's fossa, it can often be located beneath the lateral margin of the pectoralis major muscle. Less commonly, it is found bordering the deltoid muscle. In very athletic individuals or in those with

R. Hennes (ed.), *Port Surgery*, https://doi.org/10.1007/978-3-662-70624-4_6

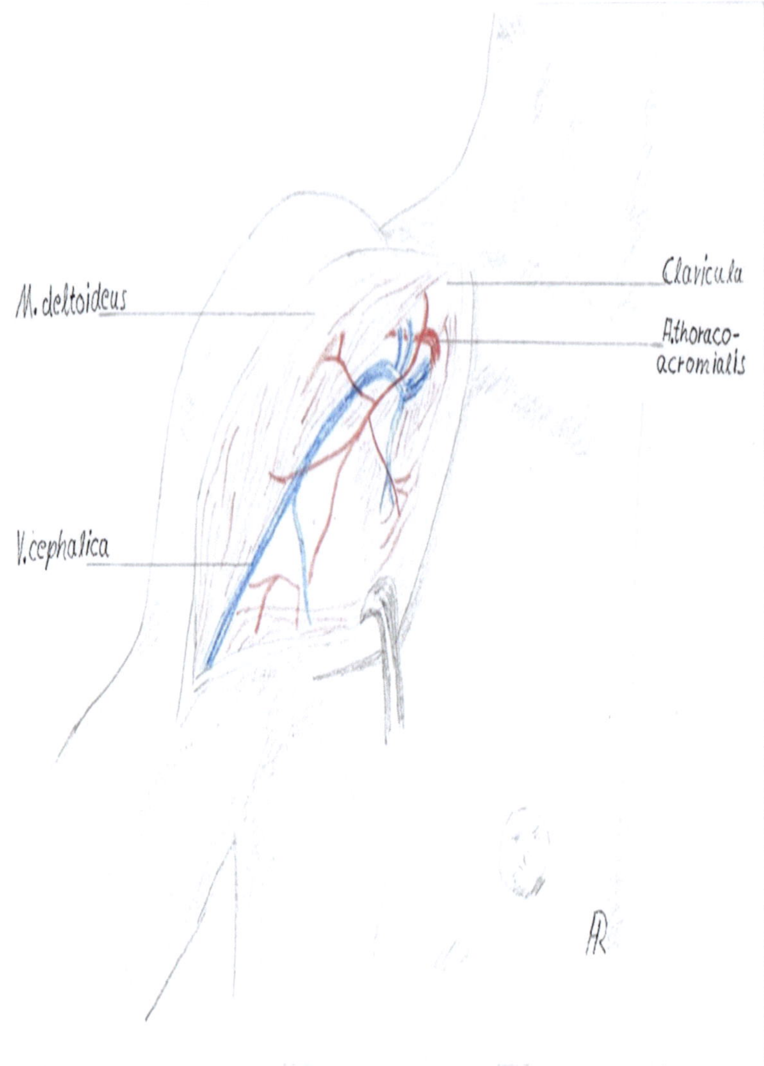

Fig. 6.1 Illustration of Mohrenheim's fossa with visualization of the cephalic vein. (© R. Hennes; all rights reserved)

a highly developed pectoralis major and deltoid muscle, the typical anatomy of Mohrenheim's fossa as described above may be altered.

The pectoralis major muscle transitions directly into the deltoid muscle, making Mohrenheim's fossa indistinguishable.

In such cases, the approach should be guided by the medial margin of the humeral head and the orientation of the muscle fibers. Generally, the fiber direction of the deltoid muscle can be clearly distinguished from that of the pectoralis major. The cephalic vein can then be exposed by longitudinal retraction of the pectoralis major and deltoid muscles. Generally, Mohrenheim's fossa and the cephalic vein become clearly visible at this stage. This incision also provides excellent access for puncture of the subclavian vein. If the incision is made as described, approximately one fingerbreadth below the clavicle over Mohrenheim's fossa, puncture of the subclavian vein through this incision is straightforward.

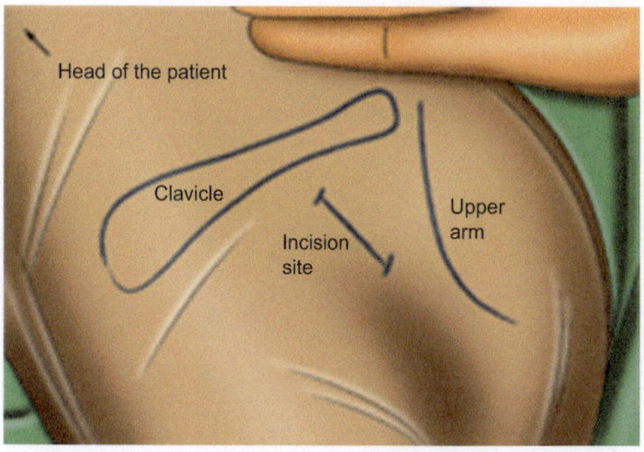

Fig. 6.2 Surgical planning of the access route to the cephalic vein in Mohrenheim's fossa. (© R. Hennes; all rights reserved)

2) Lateral cervical triangle—access to the internal and external jugular veins

As shown in Fig. 6.3, the external jugular vein lies superficially over the sternocleidomastoid muscle and, if of sufficient caliber, is easily accessible for puncture as well as for open venous cutdown. Figure 6.4 shows the intraoperative exposure of the external jugular vein.

The internal jugular vein is easily accessible medially via the anterior border of the sternocleidomastoid muscle at the level of the cricoid cartilage. For lateral access, venous cutdown or puncture can be performed at the posterior border of the muscle at the crossing point with the external jugular vein.

3) Superficial and deep neurovascular structures in the femoral triangle of the inguinal region

In Fig. 6.5, the superficial and deep neurovascular structures in the femoral triangle and inguinal region are shown. In the inguinal region below the inguinal ligament, there are several options for accessing the femoral vein and thus the inferior vena cava. For example, access can be obtained via the great saphenous vein, through smaller veins draining into the femoral

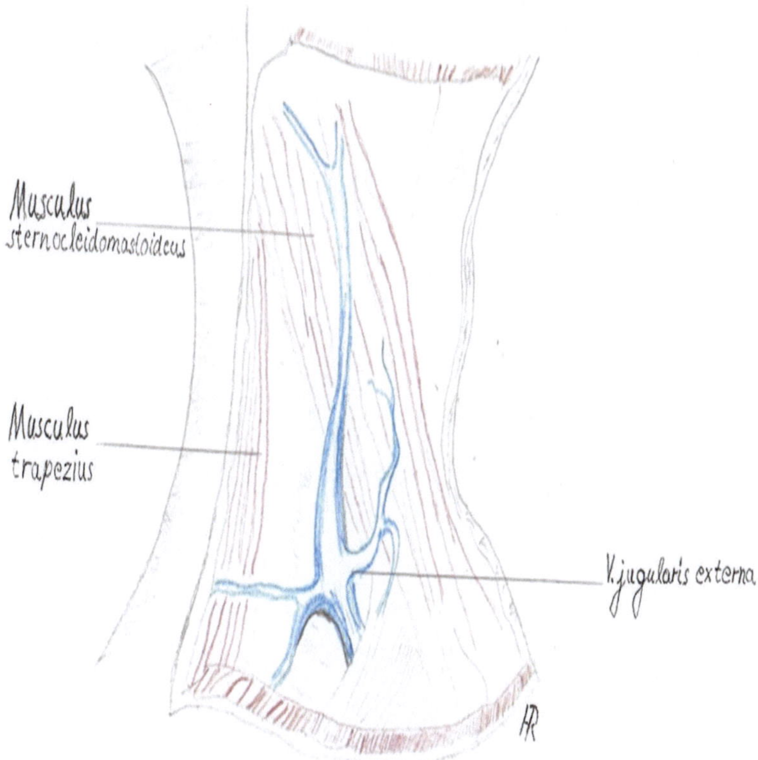

Fig. 6.3 Lateral cervical triangle with visualization of the external jugular vein. (© R. Hennes; all rights reserved)

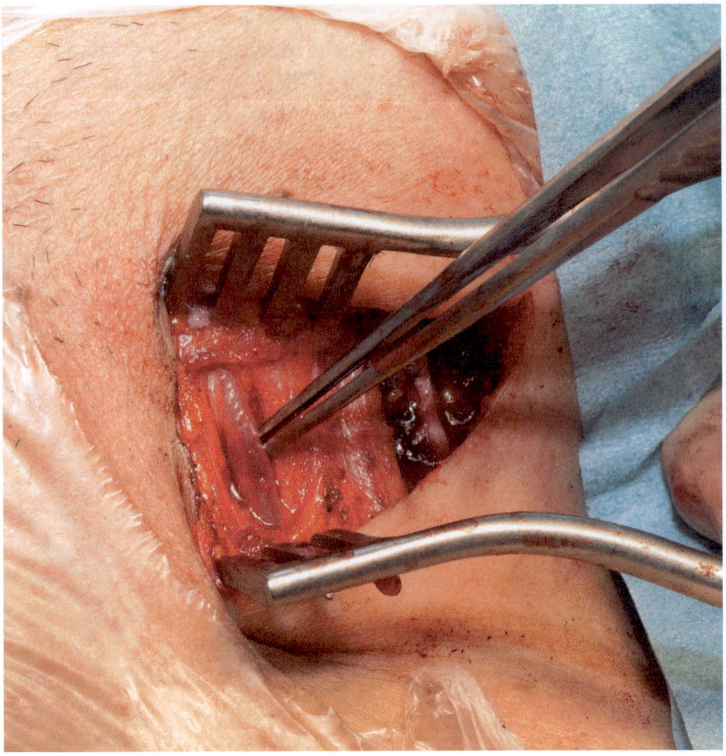

Fig. 6.4 Access to the right side of the neck via a transverse incision with visualization of the external jugular vein. (© R. Hennes; all rights reserved)

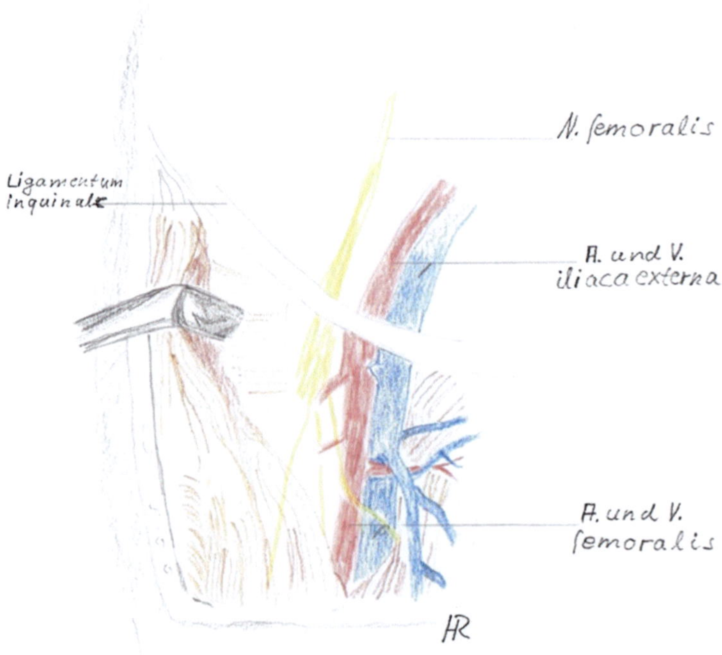

Fig. 6.5 Neurovascular structures of the right femoral triangle. (© R. Hennes; all rights reserved)

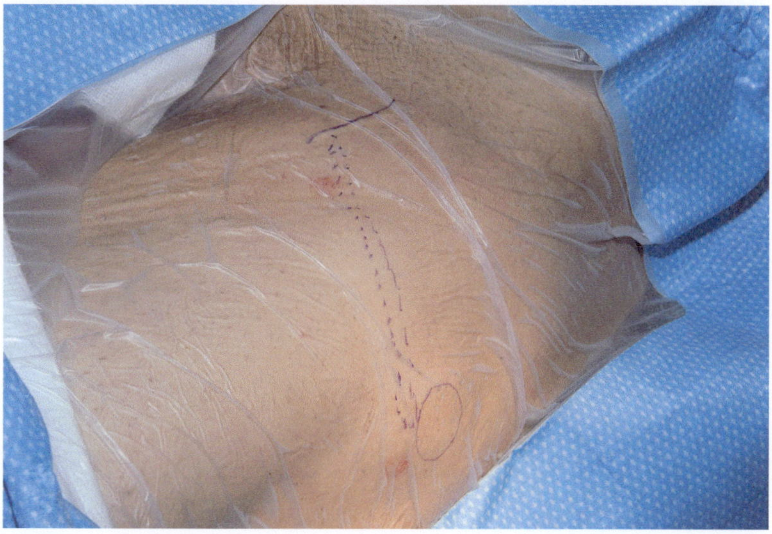

Fig. 6.6 Planned incision in the left groin with planned tunneling and port chamber placement. (© R. Hennes; all rights reserved)

vein, or by direct puncture of the femoral vein below the inguinal ligament.

Surgical planning of the incision in the groin, including tunneling and port chamber placement, is shown in Fig. 6.6.

Reference

Tillmann BN (2016) Atlas der Anatomie. Springer

7 Perioperative Hygiene in Port Procedures

Alexander Daniel Wollkopf and Vanessa Eichel

▶ Infections of the port system are a feared complication and often lead to explantation of the device. Patients frequently present with numerous predisposing risk factors, such as immunosuppression and malignant tumors. The majority of these nosocomial wound infections can be prevented through appropriate preventive measures. The hands of healthcare personnel serve as a principal route for pathogen transmission. Nevertheless, instrument reprocessing and skin antisepsis are integral elements of a comprehensive hygiene strategy. Based on the current national and international guidelines, the following section outlines evidence-based perioperative hygiene measures.

7.1 Fundamentals of Hygiene

Approximately one quarter of nosocomial infections manifest as postoperative wound infections, representing a particularly feared complication after port implantation (Behnke et al. 2017). In adult patients, about 4.6% of implanted ports are associated with device-related sepsis, and in children, the rate is as high as 16.3% (Jiang et al. 2020). Once a port becomes infected, eradication is difficult, necessitating explantation in approximately 80% of cases (Vidal et al. 2016). This is associated with significantly increased morbidity, additional interventions, prolonged hospitalization, reduced quality of life, and considerable additional costs for the healthcare system (Badia et al. 2017; Lebeaux et al. 2012).

Infection of the port system can occur via the following routes:

- Endogenously through
  - Skin flora in the surgical area
  - The patient's own flora outside the surgical area
  - Hematogenous dissemination from a distant infectious focus, resulting in septic embolization at the catheter site
- Exogenously through
  - Flora of healthcare personnel, especially hands and droplets
  - Contaminated instruments, port systems, consumables (port needles, infusions, syringes, etc.)

Clinically, port infections may present as localized postoperative wound infections or as

A. D. Wollkopf (✉)
Institut für Hygiene und Public Health, Universitätsklinikum Bonn, Bonn, Germany
e-mail: alexander.wollkopf@ukbonn.de

V. Eichel
Sektion für Krankenhaus-und Umwelthygiene, Zentrum für Infektiologie, Universitätsklinikum Heidelberg, Heidelberg, Germany
e-mail: vanessa.eichel@med.uni-heidelberg.de

R. Hennes (ed.), *Port Surgery*, https://doi.org/10.1007/978-3-662-70624-4_7

vascular catheter-related bloodstream infections. (with bacteremia, recurrent fever episodes after port use, etc.). While local wound infections affect about 33% of patients, port system infections more commonly present in the systemic form, frequently confirmed by pathogen isolation from port chamber aspirates and/or peripheral blood cultures (Vidal et al. 2016).

Approximately one to two thirds of all postoperative wound infections are considered avoidable if appropriate preventive measures are implemented (Umscheid et al. 2011). This underscores the great potential and critical importance of infection prevention and hygiene measures in both placement and ongoing management of port systems.

7.2 Recommendations of Professional Societies

The recommendations in this chapter are based—alongside legal requirements such as TRBA 250—on the current guidelines of the Commission for Hospital Hygiene and Infection Prevention (KRINKO), the Centers for Disease Control and Prevention (CDC), the Society for Healthcare Epidemiology of America (SHEA), the Infectious Diseases Society of America (IDSA), the National Institute for Health and Care Excellence (NICE), the World Health Organization (WHO), and the American College of Surgeons and Surgical Infection Society (ACS-SIS).

7.3 Hand Hygiene

The hands of medical personnel play a major role in the transmission of nosocomial infections, making consistent hand hygiene critically important. Without appropriate measures, they serve as a significant reservoir and primary vehicle for the transmission of nosocomial pathogens.

Therefore, hands and forearms must remain uncovered and readily accessible for effective disinfection at all times. All jewelry, including rings and bracelets, must be removed prior to commencing work. Fingernails should be kept short, unpolished, and natural, without the use of artificial nails or nail enhancements.

Hand Washing

Hands should be washed before starting work, after using the restroom, when visibly soiled, and optionally at the end of the workday. For invasive procedures that require surgical hand disinfection, the forearms up to and including the elbows should also be washed. This effectively removes gross contamination and bacterial spores, which are not sufficiently inactivated by standard hand disinfectants. Except for heavy soiling of the fingernails, the use of brushes is no longer recommended, as the resulting microlesions in the skin promote microbial colonization.

This allows the hands to dry thoroughly and prevents dilution of the disinfectant.

Hygienic Hand Disinfection

A distinction exists between hygienic and surgical hand disinfection. Surgical hand disinfection, applied prior to invasive and aseptic procedures, is more intensive and comprehensive (see Sect. "7.7 Peri- and Intraoperative").

(follow manufacturer's instructions). Critical and often inadequately disinfected areas include the thumbs, fingertips, nail folds, and interdigital spaces, which should receive special attention. Although there is no single "correct" rubbing technique, a standardized approach facilitates training of new staff. It is essential that all areas of the hands are thoroughly covered with disinfectant throughout the process.

The WHO has defined "5 Moments for Hand Hygiene" when hygienic hand disinfection should be performed:

1. Before patient contact
2. Before aseptic procedures

3. After contact with (potentially) infectious material
4. After contact with the patient
5. After contact with the immediate patient environment (e.g., bed, bedside table, all devices belonging to the patient)

In addition, hand disinfection must always be performed after removing disposable gloves (Fig. 7.1).

If hands are visibly contaminated, the contamination should be removed with a paper towel soaked in disinfectant or similar, followed by standard hand disinfection. If hand washing is required, it should be performed only after the disinfectant's designated contact time has fully elapsed.

Skin Protection/Care

In patient care, hands of medical personnel are subjected to significant stress (e.g., due to the moist skin environment when wearing gloves). Therefore, regular application of skin protection products to the hands is essential. This measure should not be underestimated, as only intact skin permits effective disinfection. Like any precision instrument, hands require consistent care to maintain functionality.

> **Practical Tip** The most important preventive measure is correct hand hygiene. Make sure to integrate this consistently into your daily workflow.

7.4 Rooms and Facilities

Rooms

Depending on the type of procedure and the risk of infection, different requirements are placed on the facilities. Port implantations are classified as "operations," which—unlike "procedures"—require full compliance with the standards of an operating room (Kassenärztliche Vereinigung Bayern 2017; DGKH 2021). The spatial requirements include:

- Functional separation of the operating area, including a sluice system (separate for staff, patients, clean and contaminated materials)
- Adequate room facilities:
  - In addition to the operating room, separate rooms for each of the following:
- reprocessing of used instruments or medical devices (contaminated workroom); storage of reprocessed medical devices/sterile goods;

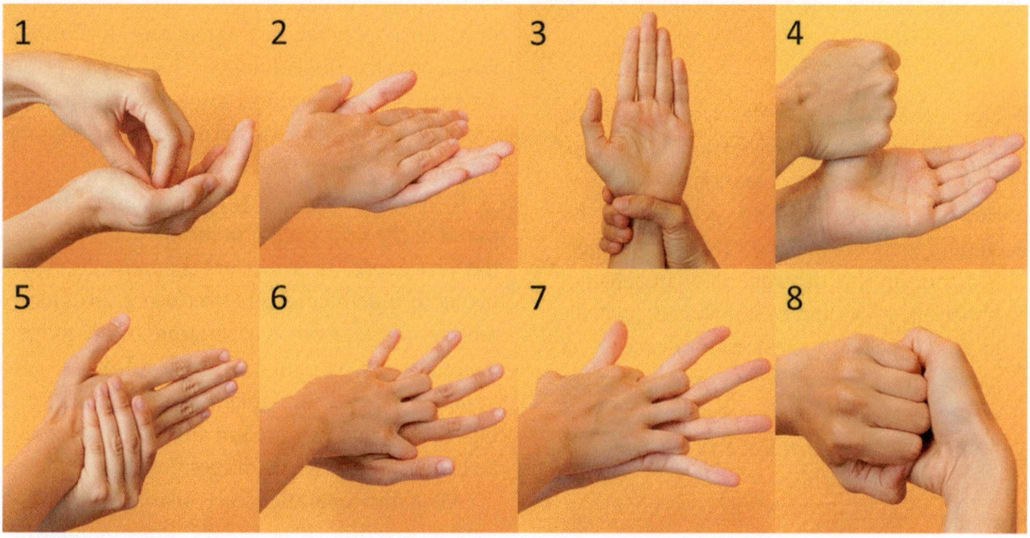

Fig. 7.1 Procedure for surgical hand disinfection. (Courtesy of © Alexander Wollkopf and Vanessa Eichel [2021].)

storage of cleaning supplies; office space; staff lounge
  - Areas *or* rooms for:
- anesthesia induction/patient preparation; postoperative monitoring; surgical hand disinfection/hand hygiene
  - If necessary, a preparation room for instrument tables, and if needed, a patient changing room
  - Staff sluice with: clean and contaminated sides, areas/cabinets for ward clothing, laundry bag for used clothing, washbasin, toilet, if necessary, shower, protected storage areas for clean area clothing, disinfectant dispenser
- Adequate room air quality:
  - For operating rooms and preparation rooms for instrument setup, triple-filtered air according to room air class Ia or Ib (i.e., supply air filter class H13 on the room side, exhaust air filter at least class M5, low-turbulence displacement ventilation for Ia, or turbulent mixed ventilation for Ib)
  - Additionally, positive pressure ventilation in the operating room to prevent the ingress of particles or pathogens from adjacent rooms
  - Window ventilation is unsuitable for operating rooms due to the absence of supply air filtration

▶ **Practical Tip** In day-to-day clinical practice, you will rarely be involved in the conceptual design of your operating department. However, good planning is essential for smooth workflows. From a hygiene perspective, the aim is to separate different activities (especially clean and contaminated) spatially or functionally to prevent transmission of pathogens. When planning renovations or new construction, it is advisable to involve hospital hygiene experts at an early stage.

Surfaces

Patient-adjacent surfaces, work surfaces, furnishings, walls, and floors must be smooth, seamless, and resistant to cleaning and disinfecting agents. The following must be disinfected:

- All work surfaces before aseptic procedures
- After each operation: patient-adjacentt surfaces, visibly contaminated surfaces, and the floor of the operating room
- At the end of the working day: the entire operating room
- At regular intervals or in case of visible contamination: all other areas such as the scrub room, sluice, etc.

If contamination with bacterial spores or non-enveloped viruses (e.g., Clostridioides difficile, noroviruses) is suspected, a sporicidal or virucidal disinfectant must be used accordingly. The product should be listed by the RKI and/or VAH.

7.5 Instruments

Medical devices and instruments must be reprocessed properly according to clearly defined standards. The intended use and the material properties play a significant role in this process. Based on the requirements for reprocessing, a categorization is performed (see Table 7.1) with increasing demands on the reprocessing procedure. Intraoperative instruments for port implantation are classified almost exclusively as critical devices. Consequently, only properly sterilized reusable instruments or sterile single-use materials should be employed.

Instruments for port implantation are prepared in the operating room immediately prior to the procedure. In select cases, preparation may occur in a dedicated adjacent room, provided it adheres to equivalent operating room hygiene standards (in particular, it must fulfill the same ventilation and air quality requirements). If instruments are prepared in advance, they should be covered with sterile drapes until use.

After the operation, all instruments requiring sterilization (if necessary, after manual precleaning) are placed in suitable containers and transported to the reprocessing unit. It should be

Table 7.1 Classification of medical devices according to KRINKO and BfArM

Classification	Reprocessing steps	Example
Non-critical **= Contact only with intact, healthy skin**		
	Cleaning and disinfection	Stethoscope, blood pressure cuff
Semi-critical **= Contact with mucous membranes or compromised skin**		
A (without special requirements for reprocessing)	(Pre-cleaning), cleaning and disinfection, (sterilization)	Speculum, tongue depressor
B (with special requirements for reprocessing)	Pre-cleaning, cleaning, disinfection, (sterilization)	Flexible endoscopes (e.g., gastroscope), TEE probe
Critical **= Penetration of (mucous) skin, contact with blood or sterile tissues/organs, use of blood (products) and sterile drugs**		
A (without special requirements for reprocessing)	(Pre-cleaning), cleaning, disinfection, sterilization	Wound hook, forceps
B (with special requirements for reprocessing)	Pre-cleaning, cleaning, disinfection, sterilization	MIC trocar
C (with particularly high requirements for reprocessing)	Pre-cleaning, cleaning, disinfection, sterilization	ERCP catheter

ensured that used instruments do not come into contact with unused, sterile instruments (disposal/transport via the contaminated work area, no interim storage with sterile goods).

> **Practical tip** Before starting the procedure, check the instruments and materials for integrity and functionality. Ensure that they have been properly reprocessed.

7.6 Preoperative

Measures to reduce the risk of surgical site infection can be implemented even before hospital admission. Factors generally associated with an increased risk of wound infection include:

- Prolonged preoperative hospital stay
- Advanced age
- Comorbidities such as ischemic vascular disease, chronic renal insufficiency, diabetes mellitus, obesity, malignant diseases, anemia
- Previous radiotherapy
- Immunosuppression
- Malnutrition, excessive alcohol consumption, prolonged postoperative fasting
- Smoking
- Nasal *Staphylococcus aureus* colonization (risk of wound infection up to sixfold higher in orthopedic procedures)
- Existing infections in other body regions at the time of surgery

Preventive measures

- Minimizing preoperative hospital stay or planning the procedure on an outpatient basis
- Appropriate nutritional management and avoidance of prolonged fasting periods
- Normalization of blood glucose levels with a target range of 80–120 mg/dL
- Screening for and treating existing infections prior to port implantation (e.g., dental root treatment)
- Personal hygiene: Patients should bathe thoroughly the evening before or on the day of surgery, cleaning the entire skin surface including areas beyond the surgical field
- Preoperative hair removal: Should only be performed if technically necessary. In such cases, hair should be trimmed with electric clippers; shaving with a razor causes microlesions of the skin and increases the risk of infection.
- Preoperative decolonization: Always recommended in cases of MRSA colonization. Otherwise, for procedures with a high incidence of *Staphylococcus aureus*-related wound infections (especially in orthopedics and cardiac surgery), the decision should be made based on local infection rates and the prevailing spectrum of pathogens.
- Immunosuppression: Although immunosuppressive therapy is associated with an increased risk of infection, the WHO advises against interrupting therapy whenever possible due to potential side effects.
- Medium- to long-term: weight normalization, abstinence from alcohol and nicotine

7.7 Peri- and Intraoperative

In addition to standard hygiene measures, maximal barrier precautions significantly reduce the risk of infection when placing central venous catheters. This includes not only surgical hand disinfection but also wearing sterile gloves, a sterile gown, a cap, and a mask. Adequate skin antisepsis and extensive sterile draping around the surgical field are also required.

Surgical hand disinfection

Surgical hand disinfection is performed before all sterile procedures and serves to extensively inactivate the resident skin flora. It should be carried out by the entire surgical team (including instrument nurses) and must include both hands and forearms. The required exposure time depends on the disinfectant manufacturer, but is usually >90 s.

Procedure (see Fig. 7.1)**:**

1. Thoroughly rub both hands, then the forearms up to the elbows
2. Rub hands again thoroughly, paying special attention to problematic areas (nail folds, fingertips, interdigital spaces, thumbs). Keep hands completely wet throughout the entire exposure time. The amount of disinfectant used is irrelevant. Hold hands above elbow level so that any running disinfectant flows away from the hands.
3. Allow hands to dry completely. After 1 min of air drying, the disinfectant effect of alcohol-based agents is significantly improved; this also helps prevent skin irritation and glove perforation. Do not shake hands dry, as this causes the disinfectant to evaporate more quickly (and may not allow sufficient exposure time), increasing the risk of recontamination.

Gown and gloves

To protect both staff and patients, sterile disposable gowns are worn. These must be fluid-repellent/-proof and impermeable to particles (barrier function). Single sterile gloves are usually sufficient for port implantation. For infectious patients and when handling sharp-edged implants or instruments, double gloving is recommended. This provides increased personal protection; however, glove perforations are also associated with higher rates of wound infection. After surgical hand disinfection, the gown is donned first in the operating room, followed by gloves. At the end of the procedure, protective clothing is removed and disposed of in the operating room.

A typical sequence before the start of surgery might be as follows

- Wash hands with water and soap immediately upon starting the shift
- Enter the operating/procedural area: change clothes, put on cap and mask, etc.—by this time, the recommended 10-min interval between hand washing and disinfection will have elapsed
- Perform hygienic hand disinfection before entering the operating suite
- Position the patient and perform other necessary tasks
- Immediately before surgery, perform surgical hand disinfection and, only with dry hands, put on sterile gloves to carry out skin antisepsis on the patient
- Remove gloves, disinfect hands again, allow to dry, and put on a sterile surgical gown and new sterile gloves. Meanwhile, the skin antiseptic can take effect on the patient.
- From the time of surgical hand disinfection, and especially when changing gloves, take care to avoid recontamination of the patient and your own hands

Skin Antisepsis and Surgical Draping

Skin antisepsis removes or largely suppresses the patient's resident skin flora, thereby aiming to prevent contamination and infection of the implanted port system and the wound. For this purpose, the surgical area is thoroughly rubbed with a suitable skin antiseptic immediately before surgery. Alcohol-based disinfectants with the addition of a residual-effect agent (e.g., 2% chlorhexidine or 0.1% octenidine) are suitable options. Alcohol has a broad spectrum of activity and produces rapid effects, while residual-effect agents prolong and enhance efficacy. The preparation is applied generously to the surgical area—e.g., using a sterile sponge forceps and swabs. This achieves not only a chemical effect but also a mechanical removal of skin debris, including microbial pathogens. It is important not to leave any skin areas within the surgical field untreated. Colored products facilitate visualization of coverage gaps during application, ensuring complete skin antisepsis. Skin disinfectants must be allowed sufficient contact time for optimal efficacy; this duration should be extended for areas rich in sebaceous glands (refer to manufacturer's instructions).

Sterile draping is applied only after the disinfectant has completely dried. This ensures sufficient exposure time for the skin disinfectant without compromising the adhesive efficacy of the sterile drape. The exposed skin area should be kept as small as possible, and the surrounding surgical field should be covered completely with generously sized drapes. Sterile drapes must be impermeable to both particles and fluids. Incision drapes may be employed in select cases to enhance barrier integrity. These additionally cover the otherwise exposed skin area with a self-adhesive, transparent film. The skin incision is made through this film. Complete coverage is intended to reduce wound infections caused by the patient's own skin flora. Contrary to expectations, five studies encompassing 3082 surgical patients demonstrated that incision drapes increased the risk of surgical site infections(RR 1.23) (Webster and Alghamdi 2013). Another two studies using iodine-impregnated drapes found no significant difference. Accordingly, current international guidelines do not recommend the routine use of incision drapes. A recent study from Germany involving 100 patients undergoing port surgery observed no postoperative wound infections in either group and is therefore of limited significance (Scheunemann et al. 2022). Larger randomized controlled trials specifically evaluating incision drapes in port implantation surgery are therefore warranted.

Perioperative Antibiotic Prophylaxis

Perioperative antibiotic prophylaxis for port implantation has not demonstrated significant reductions in infection rates in prior studies (Johnson et al. 2016; Karanlik et al. 2011; Di Carlo et al. 2011; van de Wetering et al. 2013). Considering increasing antibiotic resistance and side effects (e.g., allergic reactions or *C. difficile*-associated diarrhea), it should thus not be used routinely.

Wound Closure and Dressing
The method of wound closure influences the risk of surgical siteinfection. The use of antimicrobial-coated suture material may be beneficial, although its value in different patient groups remains controversial. A meta-analysis on the use of triclosan-coated suture material by Ahmed et al. (2019) showed significantly reduced surgical site infection rates. In the 2018 KRINKO guideline, the recommendation for their use is "still" limited to certain patient groups (multimorbid patients, contaminated/septic surgeries, or high baseline wound infection rates), while other guidelines (WHO, CDC, ACS-SIS, and NICE) go further and generally recommend their use.

Antiseptic wound irrigation has also been discussed as an infection-preventive measure. However, a Cochrane review of 59 randomized clinical trials with a total of 14,738 patients found no significant protective effect compared to no wound irrigation (Norman et al. 2017). The majority of current guidelines therefore do not recommend this practice. The application of antimicrobial/antibiotic ointments to the closed surgical wound is also not recommended as a preventive measure.

7.8 Postoperative

The wound is dressed under sterile conditions while still in the operating room. In the absence of local complications such as bleeding, the first dressing change should be deferred until after 48 hours postoperatively. It is advisable to continue to check the wound regularly thereafter and document its condition.

Any manipulation of the port system poses a risk of contamination and must therefore be minimized. Infections of the port occur not only during implantation but more frequently during subsequent use and maintenance. Important causes include inadequate hand disinfection by staff prior to port access, insufficient skin antisepsis, contamination of the infusion system or solutions, or—less commonly—hematogenous seeding from distant infection sites.

Puncture
Prior to port system puncture, all necessary materials—including sterile gloves, Huber needle, and locking solution—are prepared and systematically arranged on a sterile field. First, the skin over the port chamber is generously disinfected with an alcohol-based skin disinfectant (plus residual-effect agent). Sufficient exposure time must be ensured. During this interval, surgical hand disinfection is performed; once hands are fully dry, sterile gloves are donned The puncture needle (pre-flushed with sterile saline) is then picked up with the right hand, while the subcutaneously placed port chamber is stabilized with the left hand. The puncture window (or corresponding skin area) should not be touched. The port chamber is then punctured vertically. Afterwards, a sterile (fixation) dressing is applied. The infusion system should be closed with a sterile disposable cap.

Port Care/Use
An unused and unaccessed port does not require dressing. Port needles have a manufacturer-specific maximum duration of use (usually about 7 days). The indication for puncture should be critically reviewed beforehand. This should also be reassessed regularly during use, e.g., daily during ward rounds.

The dressing of an accessed port system should be changed immediately if soiled or if adhesion is inadequate. The frequency of routine, regular dressing changes without specific indication does not appear (at least for non-implanted central venous catheters) to have a significant impact on infection rates (Cochrane review by 2016; Gavin et al. 2016).

Antimicrobial Lock Solution for Inactive Port Systems

The CDC guideline on preventing vascular catheter-associated infections recommends antibiotic locking solutions only for patients experiencing recurrent infections despite adherence to optimal hygiene measures.The risks of resistance development and medication side effects argue against preventive use. A review including 918 patients found that taurolidine as a lock solution, compared to non-antibiotic lock solutions, was associated with a significantly lower incidence rate of catheter-associated infections (van den Bosch et al. 2022). Suitable lock solutions for ports remain an active area of research.

References

Ahmed I, Boulton AJ, Rizvi S, Carlos W, Dickenson E, Smith NA, Reed M (2019) The use of triclosan-coated sutures to prevent surgical site infections: a systematic review and meta-analysis of the literature. BMJ Open 9(9):e029727

Anderson DJ, Podgorny K, Berrios-Torres SI, Bratzler DW, Dellinger EP, Greene L, Nyquist AC, Saiman L, Yokoe DS, Maragakis LL et al (2014) Strategies to prevent surgical site infections in acute care hospitals: 2014 update. Infect Control Hosp Epidemiol 35(6):605–627

Badia JM, Casey AL, Petrosillo N, Hudson PM, Mitchell SA, Crosby C (2017) Impact of surgical site infection on healthcare costs and patient outcomes: a systematic review in six European countries. J Hosp Infect 96(1):1–15

Ban KA, Minei JP, Laronga C, Harbrecht BG, Jensen EH, Fry DE, Itani KM, Dellinger EP, Ko CY, Duane TM (2017) American College of Surgeons and surgical Infection Society: surgical site infection guidelines, 2016 update. J Am Coll Surg 224(1):59–74

Behnke M, Aghdassi SJ, Hansen S, Diaz LAP, Gastmeier P, Piening B (2017) The prevalence of nosocomial infection and antibiotic use in german hospitals. Dtsch Arztebl Int 114(50):851–857

Berrios-Torres SI, Umscheid CA, Bratzler DW, Leas B, Stone EC, Kelz RR, Reinke CE, Morgan S, Solomkin JS, Mazuski JE et al (2017) Centers for Disease Control and Prevention guideline for the prevention of surgical site infection, 2017. JAMA Surg 152(8):784–791

van den Bosch CH, Jeremiasse B, van der Bruggen JT, Frakking FNJ, Loeffen YGT, van de Ven CP, van der Steeg AFW, Fiocco MF, van de Wetering MD, Wijnen MHWA (2022) The efficacy of taurolidine containing lock solutions for the prevention of central-venous-catheter-related bloodstream infections: a systematic review and meta-analysis. J Hosp Infect 123:143–155

Di Carlo I, Toro A, Pulvirenti E, Palermo F, Scibilia G, Cordio S (2011) Could antibiotic prophylaxis be not necessary to implant totally implantable venous access devices? Randomized prospective study. Surg Oncol 20(1):20–25

Deutsche Gesellschaft für Krankenhaushygiene (DGKH) (2015) Krankenhaushygienische Leitlinie für die Planung, Ausführung und den Betrieb von Raumlufttechnischen Anlagen in Räumen des Gesundheitswesens der Deutschen Gesellschaft für Krankenhaushygiene. Hyg Med 40–12: 519–526

Deutsche Gesellschaft für Krankenhaushygiene (DGKH) (2021) Bauliche und funktionelle Anforderungen an Eingriffsräume. Hyg Med 46:52–56

Gavin NC, Webster J, Chan RJ, Rickard CM (2016) Frequency of dressing changes for central venous access devices on catheter-related infections. Cochrane Database Syst Rev 2:CD009213

Jiang M, Li CL, Pan CQ, Yu L (2020) The risk of bloodstream infection associated with totally implantable venous access ports in cancer patient: a systematic review and meta-analysis. Support Care Cancer 28(1):361–372

Johnson E, Babb J, Sridhar D (2016) Routine antibiotic prophylaxis for totally implantable venous access device placement: meta-analysis of 2154 patients. J Vasc Interv Radiol JVIR 27(3):339–343; quiz 344

Karanlik H, Kurul S, Saip P, Unal ES, Sen F, Disci R, Topuz E (2011) The role of antibiotic prophylaxis in totally implantable venous access device placement: results of a single-center prospective randomized trial. Am J Surg 202(1):10–15

Kassenärztliche Vereinigung Bayern (2017) Liste zur Umsetzung der Bayrischen MedHygV: Maßnahmen in Einrichtungen für ambulantes Operieren

Kommission für Krankenhaushygiene und Infektionsprävention (KRINKO) beim Robert Koch-Institut (RKI) (2004) Anforderungen an die Hygiene bei der Reinigung und Desinfektion von Flächen. Bundesgesundheitsbl 47(1):51–61

Kommission für Krankenhaushygiene und Infektionsprävention (KRINKO) beim Robert Koch-Institut (RKI) und Bundesinstitut für Arzneimittel und Medizinprodukte (BfArM) (2012) Anforderungen an die Hygiene bei der Aufbereitung von Medizinprodukten. Bundesgesundheitsbl 55(10):1244–1310

Kommission für Krankenhaushygiene und Infektionsprävention (KRINKO) beim Robert Koch-Institut (RKI) (2016) Händehygiene in Einrichtungen des Gesundheitswesens. Bundesgesundheitsbl 59(9):1189–1220

Kommission für Krankenhaushygiene und Infektionsprävention (KRINKO) beim Robert Koch-Institut (RKI) (2017) Prävention von Infektionen, die von Gefäßkathetern ausgehen. Bundesgesundheitsbl 60(2):171–206

Kommission für Krankenhaushygiene und Infektionsprävention (KRINKO) beim Robert Koch-Institut (RKI) (2018) Prävention postoperativer Wundinfektionen. Bundesgesundheitsbl 61(4):448–473

Lebeaux D, Larroque B, Gellen-Dautremer J, Leflon-Guibout V, Dreyer C, Bialek S, Froissart A, Hentic O, Tessier C, Ruimy R et al (2012) Clinical outcome after a totally implantable venous access port-related infection in cancer patients: a prospective study and review of the literature. Medicine 91(6):309–318

National Institute for Health and Care Excellence (2019) Surgical site infections: prevention and treatment—NICE guideline [NG125]

Norman G, Atkinson RA, Smith TA, Rowlands C, Rithalia AD, Crosbie EJ, Dumville JC (2017) Intracavity lavage and wound irrigation for prevention of surgical site infection. Cochrane Database Syst Rev 10:CD012234

O'Grady NP, Alexander M, Burns LA, Dellinger EP, Garland J, Heard SO, Lipsett PA, Masur H, Mermel LA, Pearson ML et al (2011) Guidelines for the prevention of intravascular catheter-related infections. Clin Infect Dis Off Publ Infect Dis Soc Am 5(9):e162–193

Scheunemann S, Daenenfaust L, Langenbach MR (2022) Use of plastic adhesive skin drapes in cancer patients undergoing totally implantable vascular access port (TIVAP) placement-a randomized controlled pilot study. Langenbecks Arch Surg 407(3):1257–1262

TRBA (2018) Technische Regeln für Biologische Arbeitsstoffe im Gesundheitswesen und und in der Wohlfahrtspflege (TRBA 250) – Deutsche Gesetzliche Unfallversicherung

Umscheid CA, Mitchell MD, Doshi JA, Agarwal R, Williams K, Brennan PJ (2011) Estimating the proportion of healthcare-associated infections that are reasonably preventable and the related mortality and costs. Infect Control Hosp Epidemiol 32(2):101–114

Vidal M, Genillon JP, Forestier E, Trouiller S, Pereira B, Mrozek N, Aumeran C, Lesens O (2016) Outcome of totally implantable venous-access port-related infections. Med Mal Infect 46(1):32–38

Webster J, Alghamdi A (2013) Use of plastic adhesive drapes during surgery for preventing surgical site infection. Cochrane Database Syst Rev 2013(1):CD006353

van de Wetering MD, van Woensel JB, Lawrie TA (2013) Prophylactic antibiotics for preventing Gram positive infections associated with long-term central venous catheters in oncology patients. Cochrane Database Syst Rev 2013(11):CD003295

World Health Organisation (WHO) (2016) Global gidelines for the prevention of surgical site infection. Geneva

8 Anesthesia in Port Procedures

Karoline Bleymehl

There are various types of anesthesia management for the implantation and explantation of port systems, Hickman and Broviac catheters, as well as for their replacement or correction. In addition to conventional general anesthesia, it is possible to use local anesthetic techniques accompanied by procedural sedation and analgesia. Regardless of which anesthetic technique the patient chooses, a thorough preoperative anesthesiological evaluation and medical history is essential.

8.1 Anesthesia for Port Procedures

According to surveys from German cancer registries, more than 500,000 new cancer cases were diagnosed in 2022. Lung cancer remains the leading cause of cancer-related death among men, accounting for 24%, while breast malignancies are the most common among women, at 18%.

Studies of patient cohorts with various malignancies reveal a high prevalence of significant comorbidities, including COPD, peripheral arterial disease, cerebrovascular disorders, pre-existing cardiac conditions, diabetes, and hypertension. This comorbidity burden is attributable to both advancing patient age and direct pathophysiological associations with the underlying malignancy. For example, chronic cigarette smoking is indisputably the main risk factor for the development of lung cancer and leads to COPD in approximately 80% of all smokers in Western industrialized countries.

Advanced patient age, existing comorbidities, and the type of underlying malignancy therefore play a decisive role in the choice of anesthetic technique for port implantation.

8.2 Local Anesthetic Techniques

Port implantation procedures, with mean durations of 11–20 minutes and superficial anatomical positioning, can be performed painlessly via local anesthetic infiltration of skin and subcutaneous tissue. Especially in patients with significant pre-existing conditions, this provides an opportunity to avoid general anesthesia and its potential complications, such as difficult airway situations ("Can't intubate, can't ventilate"), hemodynamic instability, and prolonged recovery from anesthesia.

Adjunctive procedural sedation and analgesia can further contribute to pain control; in

K. Bleymehl (✉)
Klinik für Anästhesiologie, Universitätsklinikum Heidelberg, Heidelberg, Germany
e-mail: karoline.bleymehl@med.uni-heidelberg.de

R. Hennes (ed.), *Port Surgery*, https://doi.org/10.1007/978-3-662-70624-4_8

addition, immobilization of the patient improves the conditions for procedural success, and anxiolysis increases patient comfort. Perfusor-controlled administration of analgesics and sedatives is particularly suitable for this purpose.

8.2.1 Properties of Local Anesthetics

Local anesthetics are capable of interrupting neuronal signal transmission by diffusing into the interior of nerve cells and binding to the α-subunits of voltage-gated sodium channels. Essentially, their chemical structure is based on three elements: an aromatic ring connected via an ester or amide linkage to a tertiary amino group (Fig. 8.1). Local anesthetics are fundamentally amphiphilic, meaning they possess both lipophilic and hydrophilic properties. The degree of lipophilicity influences their anesthetic potency, as more lipophilic agents, among other things, penetrate membranous and axonal structures more rapidly and exhibit a higher affinity for binding to key structures. Additionally, these agents exhibit high plasma protein binding, facilitating prolonged release and thereby extending the duration of neural blockade.

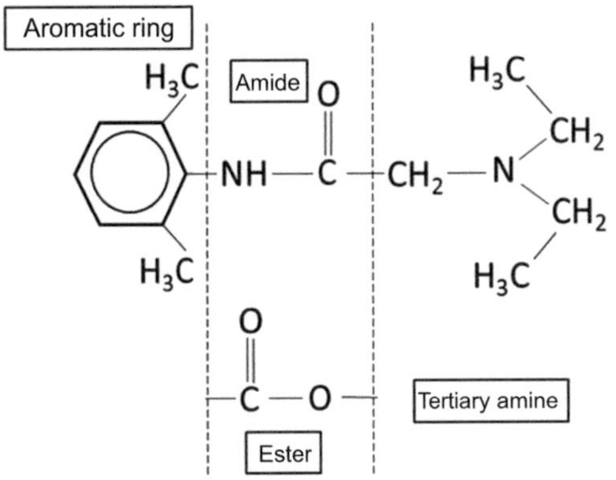

Fig. 8.1 Basic structure of local anesthetics

Since their introduction in the 1950s, amino amide local anesthetics have become established over ester-type agents, as they offer greater chemical stability and a longer duration of action. Amides exhibit lower allergenic potential, as their metabolism occurs predominantly in the liver without formation of potentially allergenic metabolites. In contemporary clinical practice, amino-amide local anesthetics are used almost exclusively.

Ideally, a local anesthetic should have a rapid onset with a long duration of action and minimal systemic side effects. Currently, depending on the type of regional anesthesia, various local anesthetics are combined to achieve these effects (Table 8.1).

Table 8.1 Properties of various amino amide local anesthetics

	Lidocaine	Prilocaine	Mepivacaine	Ropivacaine	Bupivacaine
Onset of action[1]	Rapid	Rapid	Rapid	Intermediate	Intermediate
Duration of action[1]	Short to intermediate (½–1 h)	Intermediate (1–3 h)	Intermediate (1–3 h)	Long (2–6 h)	Long (2–8 h)
Plasma protein binding rate	64%	55%	78%	95%	96%
Plasma half-life	1.6 h	1.6 h	1.9 h	1.8 h	2.7 h
t½ (min)	96	96	114	111	162
Potency	4	4	4	14	16
C_{tox} (μg/ml)	>5	>5	5–6	4	1.5

[1]Procedure/dose dependent, t½ = elimination half-life, C_{tox} (μg/ml) = systemic toxic threshold concentration

8.2.2 Toxicity

Although serious complications are rare and have shown a declining trend, they still occur with an incidence of 0.04–0.18% for peripheral regional anesthesia procedures.

The concept of an absolute maximum dose for local anesthetics warrants reconsideration, as current recommendations exhibit considerable variation and fail to incorporate pharmacokinetic data or patient-specific factors (underlying diseases, body size and weight, age). Instead, they are mainly based on a few pharmacokinetic studies and animal data extrapolated to humans. It is therefore more appropriate to adjust the dose by considering the type of regional anesthesia, the site of administration, as well as the patient's age and condition when calculating maximum doses.

It is important to note that there is no strict correlation between plasma levels of local anesthetics and the patient's body weight, meaning that systemic intoxication is possible even when maximum recommended doses are not exceeded.

After their absorption into the bloodstream, local anesthetics undergo redistribution, initially to highly perfused tissues such as the brain, heart, and kidneys, and subsequently to muscle and adipose tissue. Depending on the substance, local anesthetics bind to plasma proteins to varying degrees. The unbound fraction of the local anesthetic is fundamentally responsible for the pharmacological effect. Consequently, when high doses are used for local anesthesia, more protein binding sites are occupied and the free, active fraction increases. This is particularly relevant in the development of intoxications.

8.2.2.1 Local Anesthetic Intoxication

Local anesthetic systemic toxicity (LAST) ranks among the most serious and potentially lethal complications of local anesthetic use. Several primary forms are distinguished, differentiated by the relationship between etiology and symptom onset timing.

In the event of accidental intravenous injection, which most commonly occurs due to failure to aspirate during the administration of the local anesthetic, severe arrhythmias and central nervous system complications develop within a few circulatory cycles. Intra-arterial misinjections, on the other hand, occur more frequently during procedures in the head and neck region and lead to seizures immediately after injection; they less commonly affect the cardiovascular system. Immediate LAST manifestations result directly from inadvertent intravascular misinjection. In contrast, delayed systemic effects arise from gradual absorption of large anesthetic volumes, culminating in excessive plasma concentrations. In such cases, symptoms may appear up to 30 min after administration, depending on the plasma concentration and the proportion of unbound local anesthetic not attached to plasma proteins.

The classic sequence of LAST usually begins with central nervous system symptoms before cardiovascular effects become apparent. The central nervous system is generally more sensitive to systemically relevant plasma concentrations. However, this distinction does not always hold in clinical practice, attributable to the agents' individual properties, the administration method (e.g., infiltration versus perivascular plexus block), and diverse pharmacokinetic factors. As a result, stages may be skipped, prodromal signs may be absent, and cardiovascular symptoms may occur simultaneously or even precede neurological symptoms.

In principle, the binding affinity of local anesthetics to voltage-gated sodium channels is by no means limited to nerve cells. Essentially, any excitable cell can be affected, which is why the systemic effects can manifest in a variety of ways (Fig. 8.2).

Neuro- and Cardiotoxicity

Local anesthetics cross the blood-brain barrier and initially exert a cortical suppressive effect by inhibiting inhibitory neural circuits. Clinical

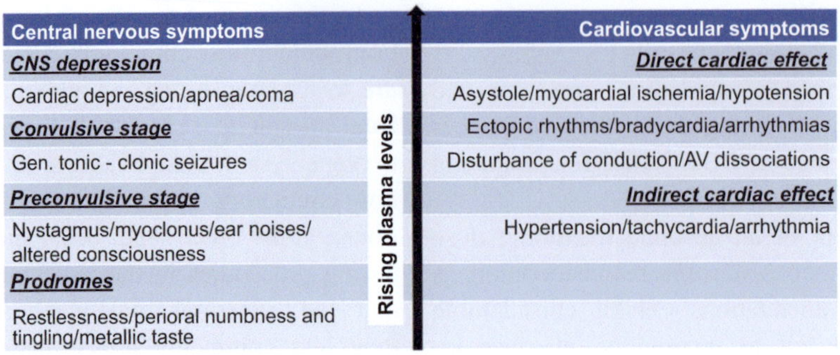

Fig. 8.2 Symptoms of LAST

symptoms such as myoclonus, tinnitus, agitation, and concentration disturbances represent uncoordinated excitatory activities that are no longer under higher-level control. Other pathognomonic signs in the prodromal stage include perioral numbness and tingling, as well as a metallic taste. Ultimately, these symptoms culminate in a tonic-clonic seizure as an expression of maximal excitation. In the final stage, further increases in plasma concentration lead to generalized cerebral depression. Untreated progression culminates in central respiratory and circulatory arrest, inevitably leading to the patient's death.

Effects on the cardiovascular system initially manifest nonspecifically as hyperdynamic states such as tachycardia and hypertension. These changes are primarily due to a centrally mediated increase in sympathetic tone. Further increases in plasma concentration, however, directly block cardiac sodium and calcium channels, causing severe arrhythmias. In particular, negative chronotropic and dromotropic effects become apparent, potentially progressing to asystole to asystole. Special attention must be paid to the substance-specific properties of local anesthetics: for example, lidocaine achieves rapid blockade by quickly entering the open sodium channel, but it also dissociates rapidly ("fast in—fast out"). In contrast, the channel blockade induced by bupivacaine resolves only slowly ("fast in—slow out"), which, in addition to other effects on cellular metabolism, confers the greatest cardiodepressive potential. Switching to less toxic derivatives such as ropivacaine is a better alternative to avoid the use of high doses of bupivacaine while achieving similarly strong and long-lasting effects. Nevertheless, due to its lipophilicity and potency, ropivacaine also possesses toxic properties.

8.2.2.2 Treatment of Intoxication and Emergency Management (Based on the Recommendations of the DGAI Professional Society)

The primary focus lies on preventing LAST events, which can be reliably avoided prior to local anesthetic procedures through targeted preventive measures. The use of regional anesthesia techniques should take place in a setting that meets the anesthesiology workplace requirements recommended by the DGAI. In addition to standard monitoring with ECG, pulse oximetry, and noninvasive blood pressure, securing the airway must always be feasible. Thus, board-certified anesthesiologists and trained support staff are indispensable. Furthermore, suitable defibrillators for cardiopulmonary resuscitation must be kept within immediate reach, and staff must be regularly trained not only in the application of CPR measures but also in the recognition and management of LA intoxications.

The administration of local anesthetics under ultrasound guidance is considered state of the art: incorrect injections and clinically significant systemic intoxications have been shown to occur less frequently. The amount of highly potent and toxic local anesthetics can also be reduced due to the more precise placement of needles compared to electrical stimulation alone or landmark-based techniques. Every injection should be performed slowly, in fractions, and with repeated negative aspirations. All involved personnel—physicians and support staff—must demonstrate proficiency in the local anesthetics, materials, and procedures employed.

To date, there is no specific medication that can truly antagonize the effects of local anesthetics or immediately reverse their action as a true antidote. Therapies for the treatment of acute intoxication are therefore more symptomatic than causal in nature. The efficacy of 20% lipid emulsion has so far been demonstrated in animal models; large, randomized, controlled studies in patients are lacking. This is partly due to the fact that severe LAST incidents are very rare. However, the early use of lipid emulsions is also emphasized by international professional societies. It should be noted that this constitutes an off-label use, but its application is well justified due to the manageable side effect profile of the solution, the potentially severe clinical courses, and the recommendations of professional societies. Every intoxication represents a serious complication that requires immediate emergency action. Various lipid emulsions are currently available on the market. Recommendations for a specific manufacturer cannot be made due to a lack of evidence for the superiority of any product. Propofol is by no means a substitute, as its fat content (1–2%) is far too low and its cardiodepressive properties are counterproductive in emergency settings. In the operating room, at least 2 × 500 ml of a 20% lipid emulsion should be stored on the emergency cart for initial treatment, with additional bottles kept within reach, as the total amount required per patient can quickly add up to 900 ml per application. Apart from severe cases requiring resuscitation and/or the initiation of eCPR/ECMO, every LAST event should be followed by appropriate monitoring. The DGAI recommends monitoring for 2 h after neurological events, such as seizures, and at least 6 h after cardiac events. These recommendations serve as guidelines and should always be tailored to the patient's condition. Further diagnostics to rule out other causes of cardiocirculatory instability or neurological deficits should be considered (see overview "Management of Intoxication").

Management of Intoxication

- **Symptoms**
  - **Cardiocirculatory:**
    - Hypertension >> Hypotension
    - Tachycardia
    - Cardiac arrhythmias
    - Conduction disturbances
    - Bradycardia/pulselessness/asystole
  - **Neurological**
    - Slurred speech
    - Metallic taste
    - Perioral numbness and tingling
    - Dizziness, tinnitus
    - Agitation, concentration difficulties
    - Excitation, seizure, coma, respiratory arrest
- **Measures**
  - **Immediate cessation of LA administration**
  - **"Call for Help"** -> initiate lipid rescue early and in parallel!
  - **Ensure oxygenation**
    - Administer oxygen, hyperventilation (acidosis increases toxic effects)
    - if necessary, intubation
- **Treat seizures**
  - Benzodiazepines i.v., e.g., lorazepam 1–2 mg i.v., midazolam 3–5 mg, repeat if necessary
  - Propofol 1–2 mg/kg, thiopental 1–5 mg/kg i.v.
  - **Note: Airway management is mandatory!**
- **Lipid rescue**
  - 20% lipid emulsion: manual bolus administration (syringe

pump—syringe) over 2–3 min (rapid administration!)
- Dosage: 100 ml for adults; for body weight <70 kg: 1.5 ml/kg
- Consider a second bolus after 5 min if symptoms persist
- Subsequently, syringe pump-controlled lipid infusion 200–250 ml over 15–20 min until the maximum dose of 12 ml/kg body weight is reached or until clinical stabilization
- Monitor for side effects!

- **Circulatory therapy**
  - Treat arrhythmias preferably with amiodarone (150–300 mg as short infusion)
  - If necessary, initiate resuscitation (ERC guidelines)
  - Resuscitation may be required for a prolonged period; consider va-ECMO in a timely manner!
  - Cautious administration of adrenaline: be aware of proarrhythmic side effects
  - Correct acidosis
  - Avoid: Ca^{2+} channel blockers/ β-blockers

8.3 Practical Procedures

Port procedures are frequently performed on an outpatient basis. However, the same standards for equipment and staffing must be applied as are customary in inpatient OR settings. To ensure structured workflows for all processes, it is advisable to develop internal SOPs and checklists. Emergency algorithms for the event of a LAST incident or anaphylactic reactions should be readily accessible at all times and regularly practiced. With regard to postoperative care, special attention should be paid to delayed-onset LAST events, allergic reactions, or surgical complications.

Outpatient procedures are often performed in remote areas, which means that additional manpower is not immediately available in an emergency. Therefore, at least specialist-level care is required for patient management.

Workflows—practical approach

- **Preoperative**
  - Comprehensive anesthesiological evaluation of the patient (“pre-anesthesia assessment”); informed consent regarding analgosedation and general anesthesia
- **On the day of surgery**
  - Ensure cardiopulmonary monitoring: ECG, NIBP, SpO2
  - Establish intravenous access: This should remain freely accessible at all times.
  - If both arms are positioned, two IV lines are required, which must be padded and routed cranially with extensions.
  - Provision of all medications and equipment according to SOP standards
  - Use of checklists according to WHO/“Team Time-Out”

8.3.1 Administration of local anesthetics

Determining a fixed dose of local anesthetic depends on various factors. The upper limits presented in Table 8.2 should serve as a guideline; however, they do not absolve medical personnel from their duty of care to respond appropriately at all times to systemic intoxication or anaphylactic reactions, as intoxications do not follow a dose-response relationship.

As previously mentioned, repeated aspirations should be performed to rule out intravascular injection, since subcutaneous infiltration for port implantation is generally guided by anatomical landmarks rather than ultrasound. With regard to anticoagulant medications, if vascular compression can be performed without difficulty and after careful risk-benefit assessment, anticoagulants do not constitute an absolute contraindication (Fig. 8.3).

Table 8.2 Maximum doses of individual local anesthetics. Limit doses for local anesthetics modified after Niesel et al., adapted to specific procedures

			Lidocaine	Prilocaine*	Mepivacaine	Ropivacaine	Bupivacaine
A	Subcutaneous injection (low blood levels)	Adults without/with adrenaline (mg/kg) Children without/with adrenaline (mg/kg)	400 mg/500 mg 6 mg/7.5 mg	600 mg 8.5 mg	400 mg/500 mg 6 mg/7.5 mg	–	150 mg 2 mg
B	Infiltration in highly vascularized regions, e.g., neck, face (high blood levels possible)	Adults (mg/kg) Children (mg/kg)	200 mg 3 mg	300 mg 4.5 mg	200 mg 3 mg	3–4 mg/kg body weight	75 mg 1 mg
C	Plexus anesthesia (increased risk of intravascular injection)	Adults without/with adrenaline (mg/kg) Children without/with adrenaline (mg/kg)	400 mg/500 mg 6 mg/7.5 mg	600 mg 8.5 mg	400 mg/500 mg 6 mg/7.5 mg	250 mg	150 mg 2 mg
D	Continuous injections (catheter placement, fractionated bolus administration)	Adults (mg/kg) Children (mg/kg)	500 mg 7.5 mg	700 mg** 10 mg	500 mg*** 7.5 mg	37.5 mg/h	200 mg 3 mg
E	Injections in highly vasoactive regions (paraspinal, epidural, sympathetic)	Adults Children	1–25 ml n/a	1–25 ml n/a	1–25 ml n/a	20–115 mg (depending on epidural technique) Children: 2–2.5 mg/kg BW	1–25 ml n/a

*Not to be used in children under 3 months (risk of methemoglobinemia)
**May accumulate after frequent and short-interval repeat doses
***No repeat dosing after this dose

Local Anesthetics for Infiltration

- Surgical skin disinfection/covering
- Subcutaneous infiltration of the surgical site with (for example):
  - Prilocaine 1% (10 mg/ml): 20–30 ml (equivalent to 200–300 mg)
  - Ropivacaine 0.5% (5 mg/ml): 10–20 ml (equivalent to 50–100 mg)
- Repeated aspiration before each injection/needle repositioning!
- If blood is aspirated: withdraw the needle, compress the puncture site

The combination of prilocaine and ropivacaine brings together the individual advantages of both local anesthetics. Prilocaine acts more rapidly than ropivacaine due to its chemical properties, while the latter has a longer duration of action. Since prilocaine is less toxic, the amount of ropivacaine can also be limited.

It should be noted that a metabolite of prilocaine, ortho-toluidine, has the ability to oxidize the divalent iron in hemoglobin to trivalent iron (methemoglobin). Normal MetHb levels in the blood are 0–2%; at 15–20%, initial symptoms such as cyanosis appear, which do not respond to O_2 administration, accompanied by dyspnea,

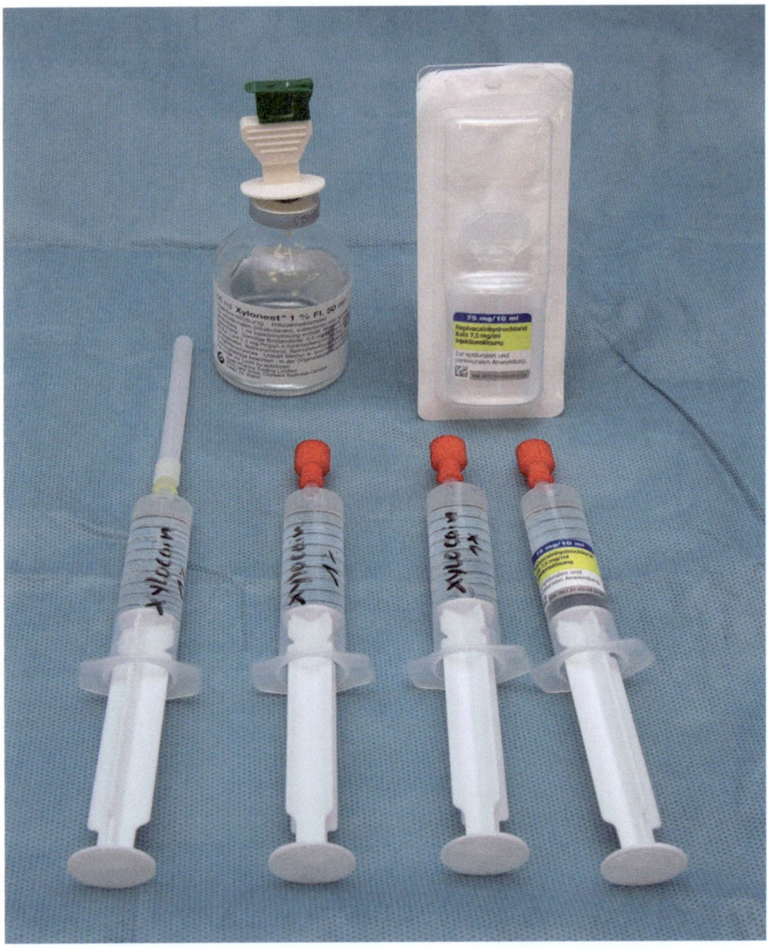

Fig. 8.3 Local anesthetics used with corresponding labeling

nausea, tachycardia, dizziness, headache, and lethargy. If such symptoms occur and a measurable increase in MetHb is detected, 2–4 mg/kg body weight of methylene blue should be administered slowly intravenously over 5 min. Side effects of too rapid injection include hypotension, arrhythmias, vomiting, and sweating. Ventricular fibrillation and asystole have been reported in rare cases. Major contraindications include glucose-6-phosphate dehydrogenase deficiency, hemolysis, and acute renal failure. For further information, please refer to the product information (Fig. 8.4).

Typically, a port procedure lasts between 10 and 30 min. Peripheral nerve blocks with ropivacaine have been shown in studies to provide analgesia for up to 10 h or more, making the use of additional medications for optimal postoperative pain control largely unnecessary.

8.3.2 Analgo-sedation

The primary aim of analgo-sedation is to increase patient comfort and to improve conditions for surgeons by preventing anxiety and stress reactions, thereby ensuring patient immobility.

In some medical fields, patients are sedated for diagnostic procedures without the presence of an anesthesiologist. In practice, analgo-sedation performed by non-anesthesiologists should be limited to mild to moderate levels of sedation in otherwise healthy patients. Midazolam has proven to be relatively safe for this purpose, as the difference between sedation and induction of general anesthesia is sufficiently large when administered cautiously and titrated, and there is ample experience with this medication. In addition, flumazenil is available as a potent antidote that can rapidly reverse its effects. The "Guideline on Sedation and Analgesia (Analgo-sedation) of Patients by Non-Anesthesiologists" issued by the DGAI in 2002 provides an overview of the relevant procedures.

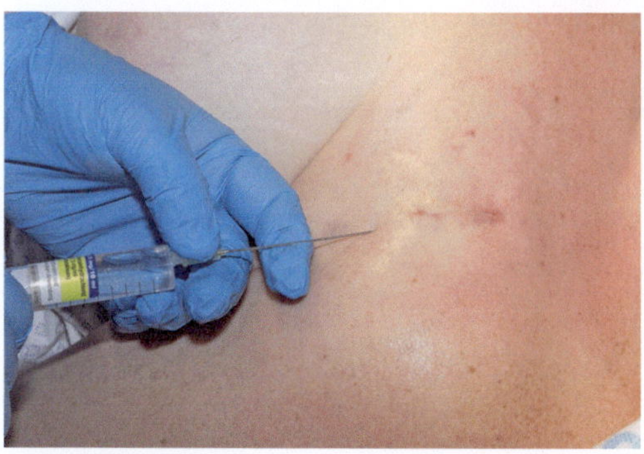

Fig. 8.4 Infiltration of the surgical site for a port replacement

The risk of severe adverse events increases significantly in inadequately supervised sedations if the following risk factors are present:

- Difficult airway conditions, e.g., tumors in the head and neck region, history of radiation therapy, space-occupying goiter, known airway difficulties, etc.
- Patients with a history of stent-PTCA, coronary artery disease, unstable angina pectoris
- Significant pulmonary diseases (COPD/asthma) with LTOT or O_2 saturation <90% on room air
- Heart failure NYHA > II
- Obesity (BMI >35 kg/m^2)
- OSAS
- Allergies or other contraindications to sedatives/analgesics
- Improper handling of hypnotics/opioids (propofol, fentanyl, etc.)

If any of the above risk factors are present, it is generally recommended that analgo-sedation be performed by anesthesiologists. This is especially true for the use of hypnotics (propofol) and/or opioids such as sufentanil, fentanyl, or remifentanil, as serious complications with life-threatening courses can occur at any time during the use of these substances. Depending on the depth of sedation, loss of protective reflexes increases the risk of aspiration; in addition, airway insufficiency may result, which is why the ability to initiate general anesthesia with airway management must always be ensured. An overview of sedation depths and the associated impairments is provided in Table 8.3. It should always be noted that the stages are fluid and that patients' physiological responses to sedatives and analgesics are subject to a wide range of influences, which cannot always be precisely predicted in advance.

Every analgo-sedation should be preceded by thorough patient counseling, which, in the sense of an anesthesiological premedication interview, includes a comprehensive medical history, medication history, questions about previous anesthetics and allergies, and, in the event of complications, the necessity of general anesthesia with airway management. Therefore, the same fasting guidelines apply as for general anesthesia. On the topic of "Analgo-sedation for diagnostic and therapeutic procedures in adults," the BDA issued a resolution in 2010 that provides information on procedures regarding analgo-sedation.

8.4 Conclusion

The most common indication for port placement surgery is malignant disease, in which chemotherapy agents must be administered. Since patients with neoplasms often suffer from potentially severe underlying conditions (cardiovascular or respiratory diseases), performing port implantation under local anesthesia is advisable to avoid the strain of general anesthesia. Another advantage of the local anesthesia-based approach is the reduction in process times and a significant decrease in costs. Comprehensive patient education from both the surgical and anesthesiological perspectives is essential. Proficiency in the use of local anesthetics, including their side effects and complications, is a prerequisite for successful outcomes; the surgical/anesthesiological setting should be equivalent to that of inpatient surgical care. Regular participation in emergency drills by all involved parties, along with the implementation of SOPs and algorithms, is standard practice. To prevent serious complications during procedural sedation, interdisciplinary collaboration between anesthesiologists and surgeons is required.

Table 8.3 Sedation stages

Sedation stages				
	Minimal sedation	Moderate sedation	Deep sedation	Anesthesia
Alertness	Normal response to verbal stimulation	Purposeful response/verbal reply to verbal or light tactile stimulation Patient can be awakened at any time	Purposeful response to painful tactile stimulation	Not arousable
Airway	Not compromised	No intervention required	Airway management may be required	Airway management required
Spontaneous breathing	Not compromised	Adequate	Impaired	Absent
Cardiovascular function	Not compromised	Usually not impaired	Usually not impaired	May be impaired
Protective reflexes	Not compromised	Preserved	Protective airway reflexes may be impaired	Abolished

References

Andreas S et al (2014) Smoking cessation in patients with COPD. Pneumologie 68(4):237–258

Becker D, Reed K (2012) Local anesthetics: review of pharmacological considerations. Anesth Prog 59(2):90–101

Baumann H, Biscoping J (2011) Toxicity of local anaesthetics-background and management. Anästh Intensivmed 52:189–198

Beck G et al (2013) Mindestanforderungen an den anästhesiologischen Arbeitsplatz Beschluss der Präsidien von BDA und DGAI am 16.11.2012 und 22.11.2012. Anästh Intensivmed 54:39–42

Čižmáriková R, Čižmárik J (2020) Chiral aspects of local anesthetics. Molecules 25(12):2738

Coburn M, Roissant R et al (2016) Qualitätsindikatoren Anästhesiologie 2015/Beschluss des Engeren Präsidiums der DGAI vom 09.11.2015 sowie des Präsidiums des BDA vom 30.11.2015. Anästh Intensivmed 57:219–230

Covino BG (1986) Pharmacology of local anaesthetics. Br J Anaesth 58:701–716

De Hert S et al (2011) Preoperative evaluation of the adult patient undergoing non-cardiac surgery: guidelines from the European Society of Anaesthesiology. Eur J Anaesthesiol 28(10):684–722

Eng HC, Ghosh SM, Chin KJ (2014) Practical use of local anesthetics in regional anesthesia. Curr Opin Anaesthesiol 27(4):382–387

Fachinformation Ropivacain-HCl-ratiopharm® 2 mg/ml / 7,5 mg/ml / 10 mg/ml Injektionslösung. Stand Oktober 2015. Rote Liste Fachinfo Service

Fowler H, Belot A et al (2020) Comorbidity prevalence among cancer patients: a population based cohort study of four cancers. BMC Cancer 20(1):2

Hemalkumar M, Sneha S et al (2018) Adapting the elixhauser comorbidity index for cancer patients. Cancer 124(9):2018–2025

Heavner JE (2007) Local anesthetics. Curr Opin Anaesthesiol 20(4):336–342

Jeffrey B, Gross MD (Chair) et al (2002) Practice guidelines for sedation and analgesia by non-anesthesiologists. American Society of Anesthesiologists. Anesthesiology 96:1004–17

Knebel P, Fischer L et al (2008) Protocol of an expertise based randomized trial comparing surgical Venae Sectio versus radiological puncture of Vena Subclavia for insertion of totally implantable access port in oncological patients. Trials 24(9):60

Lirk P, Picardi S et al (2014) Local anaesthetics: 10 essentials. Eur J Anaesthesiol 31(11):575–585

Machat S et al (2019) Complications of central venous port systems: a pictorial review. Insights Imaging 10:86

Notfall-Alghoritmus/Lokalanästhetika – Intoxikation, Empfehlung der SGAR/SSAR, basierend auf ESA-Emergency Quick Reference Guide No 09, 2012/13

Piepho T et al (2015) S1-Leitlinie Atemwegsmanagement. Anaesthesist 64:859–873

Pittiruti M, Hamilton H (2009) ESPEN guidelines on parenteral nutrition: central venous catheters. Clin Nutr 28:365–377

Robert Koch Institut. Zentrum für Krebsregisterdaten. https://www.krebsdaten.de/Krebs/SiteGlobals/Forms/Datenbankabfrage/datenbankabfrage_stufe1_form.html

Schuld J et al (2009) Venöses Portsystem. Implantation in Vollnarkose oder Lokalanästhesie? Eine retrospektive Aufwandsanalyse. Zentralbl Chir 134: 345–349

Steinfeldt T et al (2015) Wiss. Arbeitskreis Regionalanästhesie. Periphere Blockaden der oberen Extremität. Vorgehensweise Landmarken-gestützter und Ultraschall-gesteuerter Verfahren. Anästh Intensivmed 56:244–252

Taeger K (2002) Klinik für Anästhesiologie der Universität Regensburg. Leitlinie zur Sedierung und Analgesie (Analgosedierung) von Patienten durch Nicht-Anästhesisten/Beschluß des Engeren Präsidiums der DGAI vom 02.03.2002

Teichgräber UK, Pfitzmann R, Hofmann HA (2011) Central venous port systems as an integral part of chemotherapy. Dtsch Arztebl Int 108(9):147–154

Van Aken H et al (2010) Analgosedierung für diagnostische und therapeutische Maßnahmen bei Erwachsenen. Anästh Intensivmed 51:S598–S602

Verlinde M, Hollmann MW et al (2016) Local anesthetic-induced neurotoxicity. Int J Mol Sci 17(3):339

Vogelmeier C et al (2018) Guideline for the diagnosis and treatment of COPD patients-issued by the German Respiratory Society and the German Atemwegsliga in Cooperation with the Austrian Society of Pneumology. Pneumologie 72(4):253–308

Waurick K. Antikoagulantien und Regionalanästhesie – wie verfahren? DAAF Refresher Nr. 41, Düsseldorf Mai 2015

Wiesmann T et al (2019) Aus dem Wissenschaftlichen Arbeitskreis Regionalanästhesie der Dt. Gesellschaft f. Anästhesiologie und Intensivmedizin S1-Leitlinie (AWMF-Registernummer 001–044). Prävention & Therapie der systemischen Lokalanästhetika-Intoxikation (LAST). Aktualisierte Handlungsempfehlungen des Wissenschaftlichen Arbeitskreises Regionalästhesie der Deutschen Gesellschaft für Anästhesiologie und Intensivmedizin e. V. (DGAI). 05/2019

Wiesmann T, Schubert AK, Dinges HC, Wulf H, Steinfeldt T, Radke OC, Leisinger S, Eichholz R, Bünten-Hunscher B, Karst J, Döffert J (2021) S1-Leitlinie (AWMF-Registernummer 001–022): Regionalanästhesie bei ambulanten Patienten-Empfehlungen zur Durchführung. https://doi.org/10.19224/ai2021.267

Zalunardo M, Krayer S et al (2019) Swiss recommendations for non-anaesthesiologist administered procedural sedation and analgesia in adults. Cardiovasc Med 22:w02035

Zink W, Graf BM (2007) Lokalanästhetikatoxizität-Relevanz empfohlener Maximaldosen? Anästh Intensivmed 48:182–205

Zink W, Ulrich M (2018) Klinische Anwendung und Toxizität von Lokalanästhetika. Anästh Intensivmed 59:716–728. https://doi.org/10.19224/ai2018.716

9 Interdisciplinary Collaboration in the Operating Room for Port Procedures

Felix Johannes Jost

Trailer The success of the operation for the patient depends on the collaboration of the various professional groups involved. This includes not only cooperation between the operating room nursing staff and the surgeon, but also among numerous other professionals, such as anesthesia, cleaning staff, supply, and laboratory personnel. It begins with the planning of the operation and extends through to the successful postoperative care of the patient. Organizational, diagnostic, hygienic, and legal aspects must all be taken into account. Optimized collaboration ensures a significant reduction in operating time and helps prevent complications. All of this contributes to the successful care of each individual patient. Clear and unambiguous communication among the different professional groups and departments is fundamental.

9.1 Preoperative Assessments

Despite thorough planning, the execution of surgery on the day of the procedure remains subject dynamics that are often difficult to predict. Patients may forget to disclose important information, such as allergies and medications. During preoperative consultation, not all necessary questions may be asked by the clinician conducting the interview. Therefore, when the patient arrives in the operating area, it is essential to reconfirm all critical information once again. In addition, the patient's medical record should be reviewed, including verification of consent form signatures and laboratory values. Any special findings must be communicated to the surgeon without omission. For example, elevated infection markers need to be interpreted to determine whether they are tumor-related or indicate another unclear infection that would contraindicate port placement. The same applies to fever and classic signs of infection. Responsibility for performing the operation always lies with the surgeon and anesthesiologist, which is why optimal information transfer is essential. Furthermore, the urgency and timing of the first use of the port must be clarified, as patients who are about to begin therapy may benefit from immediate placement of a port catheter.

9.2 Positioning

Positioning a patient presents a daily challenge for the involved team. The patient's anatomical and pathological characteristics require

F. J. Jost (✉)
Universitätsklinikum Heidelberg, Heidelberg, Germany
e-mail: felix.jost@med.uni-heidelberg.de

R. Hennes (ed.), *Port Surgery*, https://doi.org/10.1007/978-3-662-70624-4_9

individualized and tailored positioning, performed by the responsible nursing staff in collaboration with the surgeon (Fig. 9.3). Since positioning occurs as part of the procedure, the surgeon bears primary responsibility.

Overview

Many oncology patients have comorbidities that complicate optimal positioning. These include conditions such as:

- Ascites
- Chronic pain
- Spinal fusions and metastases
- Tumors in the neck, head, and thorax
- Tracheostomy (Fig. 9.1)
- Stroke
- Paralysis

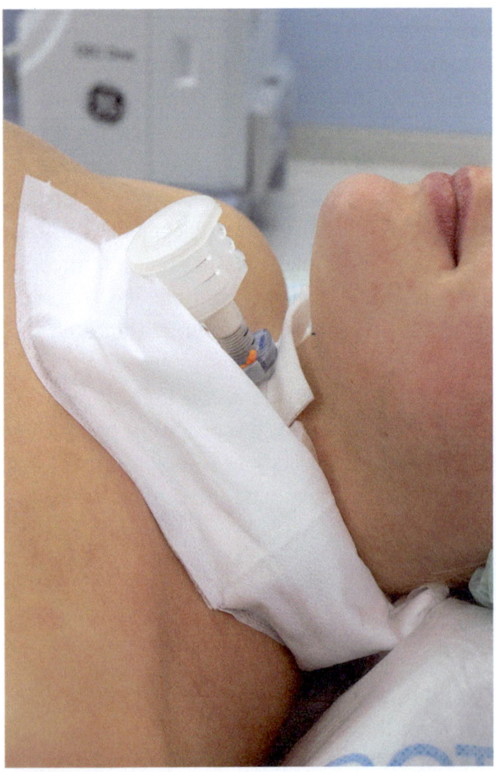

Fig. 9.1 Securing a tracheal cannula while prepping the surgical site

In addition to protecting tissues and nerves, it is essential to keep the patient still during the operation. Microsurgical procedures are particularly vulnerable to patient movement and may need to be aborted to protect the patient and ensure the procedure's success. Often, simply placing a cushion under the knees for back pain or elevating the upper body slightly in cases of dyspnea helps prevent movement. Involvement of the surgeon is indispensable in these considerations.

Positioning must never compromise the feasibility of the operation. The C-arm for intraoperative radiographic control of catheter placement must have sufficient freedom of movement to allow clear imaging of all relevant areas. Arm boards, anesthesia frames, and other positioning materials must not impede the movement of the radiographic C-arm (Fig. 9.2). Solutions should be developed collaboratively among the surgeon, operating room staff, and anesthesia team (Fig. 9.3).

9.3 Tracheostomy

A patient with a tracheostomy requires the special attention from the operating room nurse, who serves as an intermediary in the event of communication difficulties related to this artificial airway. Tracheostomized patients often have impaired verbal communication, presenting a challenge for both the surgeon and nursing staff during procedures under local anesthesia. Unlike other patients, tracheostomized patients rely on the circulating nurse's heightened attentiveness, who must manage this alongsied other intraoperative tasks Key considerations inculde ensuring a suction device is readily availabe for ongoing airway clearence. Draping should permit suctioning at any point during the procedure. Before skin prepping, protect the tracheal cannula from moisture from skin disinfectant using gauze and a securing adhesive dressing ((e.g., Fixomull® or similar; see Fig. 9.1). This should be performed proactively by the nurse. During draping, ensure the airway is not obstructed by the drapes.

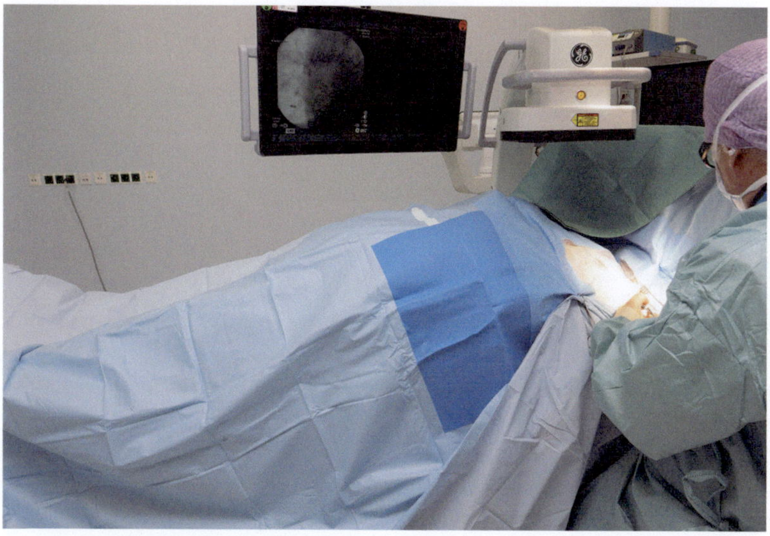

Fig. 9.2 Sterile draping and positioning of the C-arm for intraoperative imaging

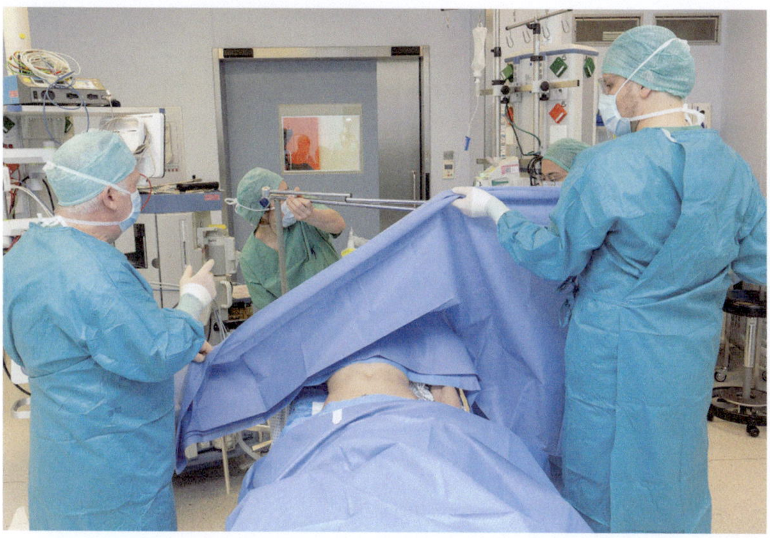

Fig. 9.3 Sterile draping of the patient as an interdisciplinary task

9.4 Anesthesia

For procedures under general anesthesia, several factors must be considered to maintain proper conduct. Distinguish among the different types of general anesthesia. Intubation anesthesia with an endotracheal tube provides optimal conditions for head positioning and mobilization, enabling proper sterile draping and maximal surgical access (see Chap. 8, Anesthesia for Port Procedures). If ventilation is provided via a laryngeal mask airway, additional securing may be required to prevent displacement and ventilation leaks during patient or drape manipulation. For procedural sedation, ensure adequate depth of sedation so the patient does not respond suddenly to painful stimuli. This is particularly important during venous cannulation or subclavian vein puncture. To optimize radiographic imaging, place monitoring cables outside the radiation field, and position ECG leads as needed. Verify the correct ECG lead placement after prepping the surgical site and correct any detachment of electrodes.

9.5 Radiation Protection

During the procedure, correctly adjusting fluoroscopy (see Fig. 9.2) is essential for accurate, clear catheter visualization while minimizing radiation exposure. X-ray use is an intraoperative task that may be delegated to a qualified nurse by an authorized, qualified physician under the Radiation Protection Act and Ordinance requirements (§ 83 RPA; § 145 Abs. 1 No. 1 StrlSchV). Strict adherence to radiation protection principles for patients and staff is mandatory. Operating room doors during the procedure for hygiene and radiation safety. All OR staff in the must wear appropriate radiation protection, including a lead apron, thyroid shield, and protective eyewear. While a thyroid shield and leaded glasses are not legally required, they are recommended (see Fig. 9.4). The surgeon, exposed to the highest radiation levels, should use this protection consistently. Maintain distance and minimize exposure to the necessary levels at all times.

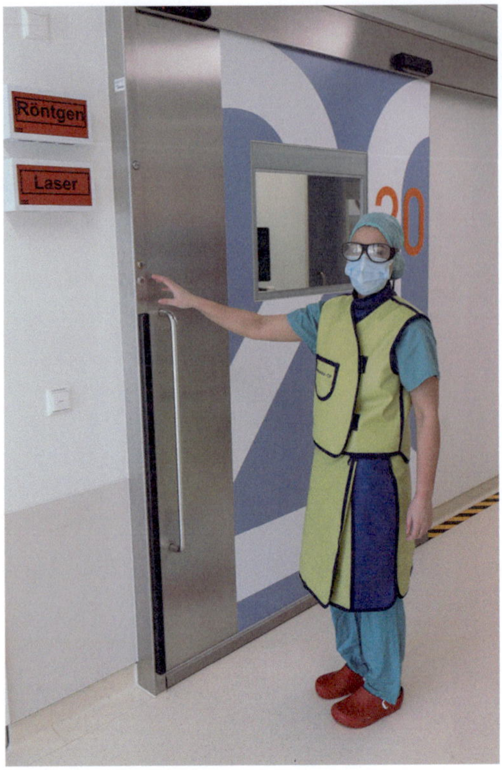

Fig. 9.4 OR staff wearing radiation protection equipment as recommended by the Radiation Protection Ordinance

References

Appelhoff B, Moser L (2020) Intraoperative und Postoperative Betreuung von Portpatienten. In: Hennes R (Hrsg) Portpflege, 1. Aufl. Springer, Berlin, S 61–66

Fantl B (2020) Wundversorgung und Verbandswechsel. In: Hennes R (Hrsg) Portpflege, 1 Aufl. Springer, Berlin, S 51–60

Hennes R, Hofmann F (2016) Ports. Springer

Hausinterner Expertenstandart zur Behandlung von Portpatienten sowie SOPs zur Operativen Versorgung am Universitätsklinikum Heidelberg

Part III

Implantation Techniques for Primary Intervention

10 Implantation of a Port Catheter via Venous Section

Roland Hennes

The venous port catheter system implanted via venous cutdown of the cephalic vein is, based on evidence, the safest implantation technique and the most favorable for patient quality of life (Hüttner et al., 2019). In approximately 94% of patients, the cephalic vein is present in adequate form and size, making it the preferred site for port catheter implantation (Knebel et al., 2011). With proper planning and incision, an experienced surgeon can typically achieve an operative time of 10–20 minutes. Intraoperative complications are rare, and cosmetic outcomes are excellent. Serious complications are not associated with this technique; pneumothorax or hemothorax cannot occur when the port is placed via the cephalic vein. The learning curve for the venous cutdown technique is straightforward, with clearly structured steps that yield very good patient outcomes.

Supplementary Information The online version contains supplementary material available at https://doi.org/10.1007/978-3-662-70624-4_10. The videos can be accessed individually by clicking the DOI link in the accompanying figure caption or by scanning this link with the SN More Media App.

R. Hennes (✉)
Klinik für Allgemein-, Viszeral- und Transplantationschirurgie, Universitätsklinikum Heidelberg, Heidelberg, Germany
e-mail: Roland.Hennes@med.uni-heidelberg.de

10.1 Introduction

The requirements for port system implantation have increased in recent years for patients in both oncology and clinical nutrition. Patients expect a safe procedure with minimal complications and the option for outpatient surgery whenever feasible. Concomitant vascular diseases, thromboses, thoracic procedures, and allergies to local anesthetics represent common challenges faced by surgeons. This raises the question of what constitutes an ideal implantation technique—one that minimizes patient burden, reduces complications, and ensures safe and efficient execution. Patient's quality of life, and especially their freedom of movement, should be restricted by the procedure as little as possible. Based on a randomized prospective study comparing open venous cutdown with puncture of the subclavian vein (Hüttner et al. 2019), Hüttner demonstrated venous cutdown of the cephalic vein to be the safest method for port catheter placement. Specific complications such as pneumothorax or hemothorax, which may arise from vessel puncture, are eliminated when exclusively using the venous cutdown technique.

The venous cutdown technique is a well-established surgical procedure used to expose veins and ensure catheter or cannula access for patients. This technique can virtually be applied any superficial vein. For port implantation via

R. Hennes (ed.), *Port Surgery*, https://doi.org/10.1007/978-3-662-70624-4_10

the cephalic vein, studies by Knebel (Knebel et al. 2011) have shown that this vein is present in 94% of cases. The preferred site is the cephalic vein in the deltopectoral groove between the deltoid and pectoralis muscles. Accurate incision placement, directly over the deltopectoral groove toward the cephalic vein, is crucial for rapid and safe exposure (see Chap. 6). There are several anatomical landmarks that must be considered during planning. When properly identified, the vein can typically be located within 1–2 minutes of operative time. The following sections describe and discuss the planning and execution of each surgical step.

10.2 Planning

As shown in Figs. 10.1 and 10.2, the incision is planned by marking the patient, with the incision made approximately one fingerbreadth below the clavicle, above the deltopectoral groove. The location of this incision offers the advantage of easy access to the subclavian vein should puncture become nexessary. Depending on the patient's body habitus, the incision length may range from approximately 3–5 cm to allow for port implantation even in obese patients.

In Fig. 10.3, a port catheter is placed on the patient for demonstration purposes, illustrating the planned implantation route via the subclavian vein to the atrium of the heart. The operating room setup and the positioning of the scrub nurse are shown in Figs. 10.4, 10.5, and 10.6. For patient positioning and instrumentation, it is important that the patient's shoulder is as close as possible to the edge of the operating table and lies flat on the table. It is often observed that patients, due to tension and anxiety, elevate their

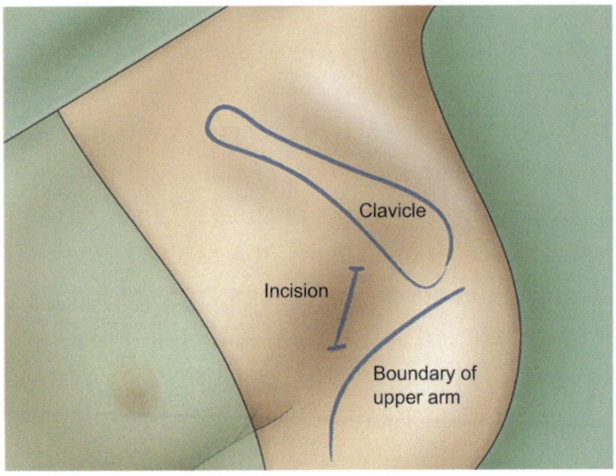

Fig. 10.1 Planning the incision. (Source Xope, © Deutscher Ärzte-Verlag; all rights reserved)

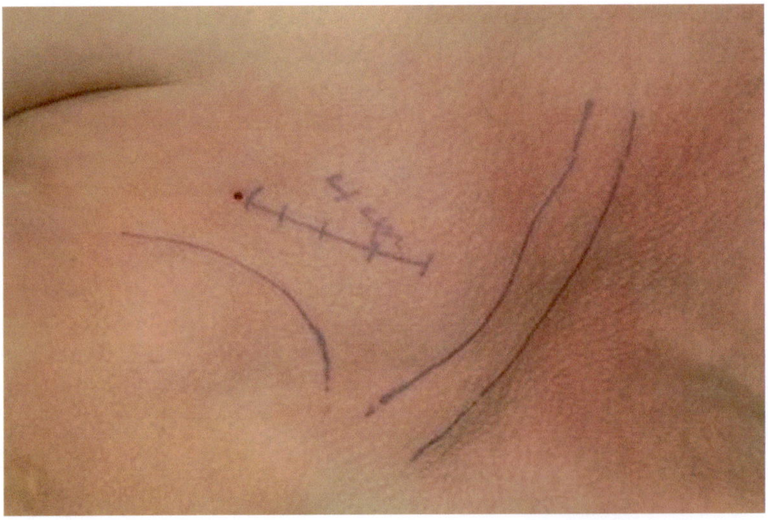

Fig. 10.2 Marking the patient for incision planning. (© R. Hennes; all rights reserved)

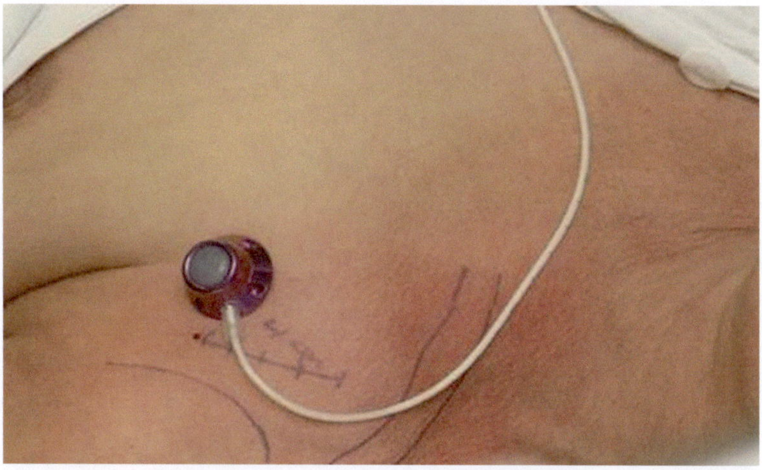

Fig. 10.3 Placement of a port catheter on the patient to demonstrate the planned position of the port chamber and catheter. (© R. Hennes; all rights reserved)

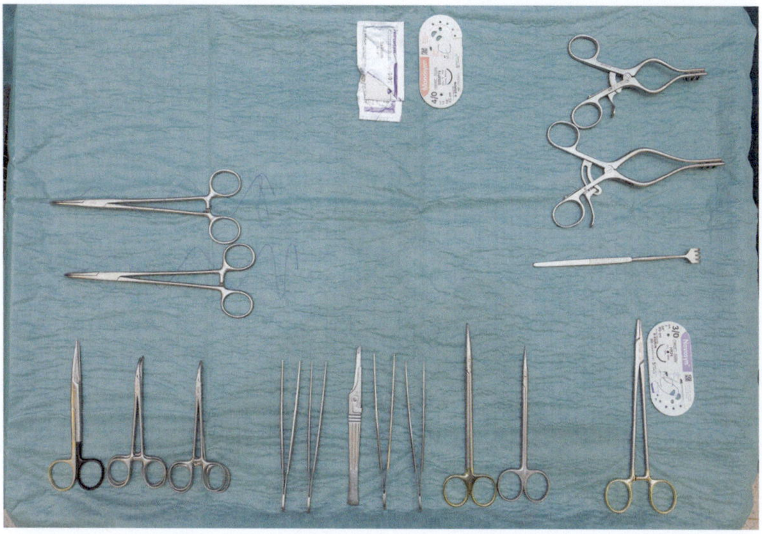

Fig. 10.4 OR setup and instruments for standardized port implantation. (© R. Hennes; all rights reserved)

shoulder, which can hinder access to the deltopectoral groove.

> **Practical Tip** At the Port Center in Heidelberg, it has proven effective over the past 15 years for the scrub nurse to stand on the same side as the surgeon, allowing for efficient instrumentation and assistance. When the procedure is performed with an assistant for training purposes, the scrub nurse can position themselves between the two surgeons. (see Fig. 10.6)..

After making the incision (see Fig. 10.7), the superficial subcutaneous tissue is divided. It has proven useful to use self-retaining retractors at this stage (see Fig. 10.8).

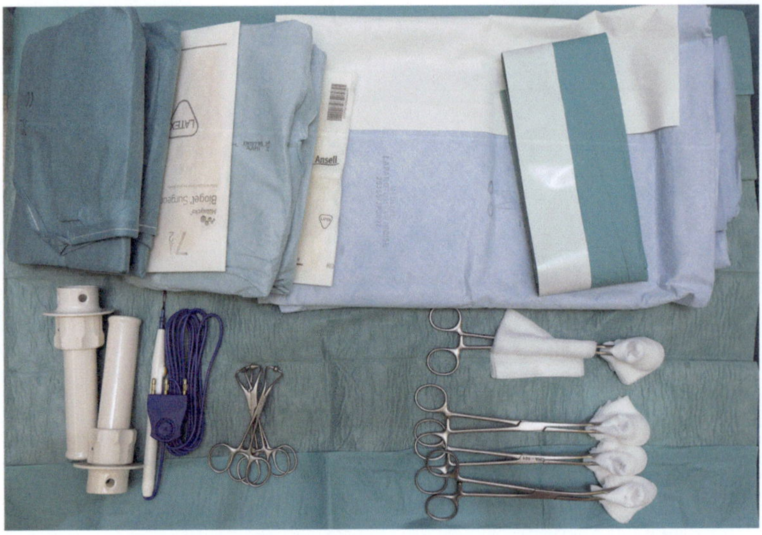

Fig. 10.5 Sterile drape, surgical gown, electrocautery, etc. (© R. Hennes; all rights reserved)

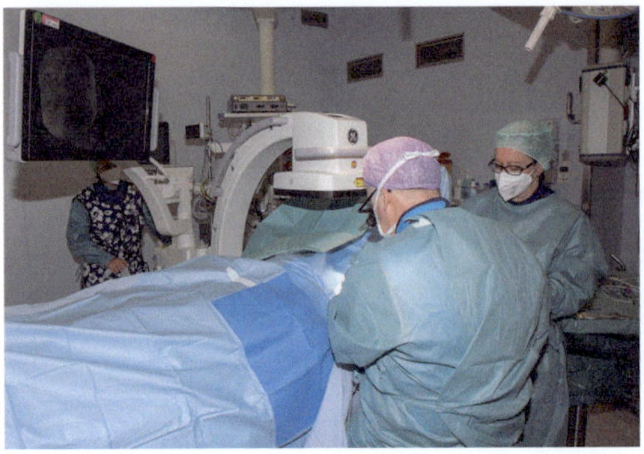

Fig. 10.6 OR setup: scrub nurse positioned on the same side as the surgeon for instrumentation and assistance.

10.3 Subcutaneous Preparation, Identification of the Cephalic Vein, Venotomy, and Insertion of the Port Catheter

After dividing the entire subcutaneous tissue, the edge of the deltoid muscle and the pectoralis muscle are exposed in order to clearly identify the deltopectoral groove. Typically, a layer of fatty fascia is encountered here, which must be incised.

Under normal anatomical conditions, the cephalic vein may subsequently be directly visualized and looped cranially and caudally (Figs. 10.9 and 10.10). This is followed by venotomy of the cephalic vein (Fig. 10.11). Depending on the size of the cephalic vein, the caudal ligature can be tied off beforehand to interrupt blood flow and improve visualization. For small veins, it is advisable to place only a clamp on the looped suture, allowing the vein to be redilated by blood flow if necessary, thereby improving visualization and access.

After the venotomy, the port catheter is inserted, ideally using forceps to guide it into the open lumen of the cephalic vein. For the venotomy technique, catheters with either tapered or rounded tips have proven effective; however, a tapered tip is generally preferred, as it facilitates smoother insertion, particularly into smaller veins. For technical reasons, tapered port catheter tips can only be manufactured from polyurethane, whereas silicone catheters can be produced only with a rounded tip (Fig. 10.12).

This is one of the reasons why we have used only polyurethane catheters for port implantation for the past 15 years(Hennes and Hofmann 2016).

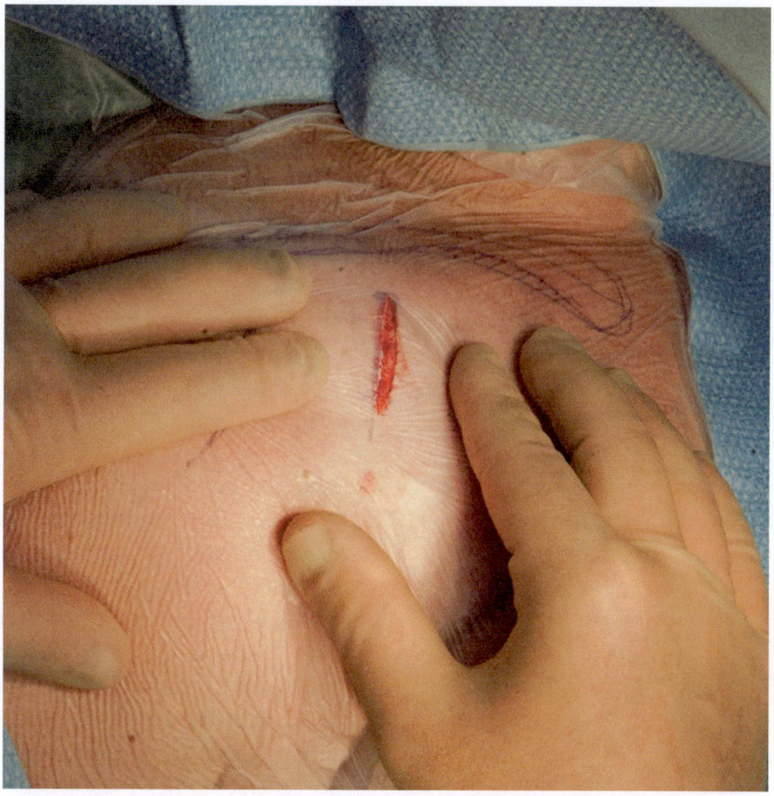

Fig. 10.7 3.5 cm incision above the deltopectoral groove. (© R. Hennes; all rights reserved)

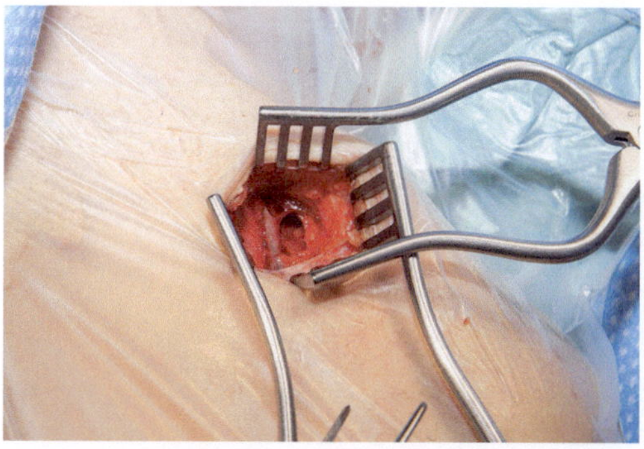

Fig. 10.8 Placement of self-retaining retractors after division of the subcutaneous tissue. (© R. Hennes; all rights reserved)

Alternatively, a vein hook—typically included in manufacturer-provided port sets—may be used. However, experience has shown that employing the vein hook often prolongs the procedure and introduces additional steps, whereas directly opening the vein with scissors and gently spreading the cephalic vein represents a faster and simpler approach. (Fig. 10.13).

Only catheters with a measuring scale, such as centimeter markings, should be used for implantation. This allows for more accurate assessment of catheter length. Based on clinical experience, catheter lengths on the left side of the thorax average approximately 20–25 cm, and on the right side approximately 15–18 cm (Fig. 10.14). These measurements depend on the patient's body habitus and height. If deviations exceeding 5–10 cm from expected measurements occur, potential causes include catheter looping or malposition. This can be readily assessed and corrected intraoperatively using fluoroscopic guidance with an image intensifier.

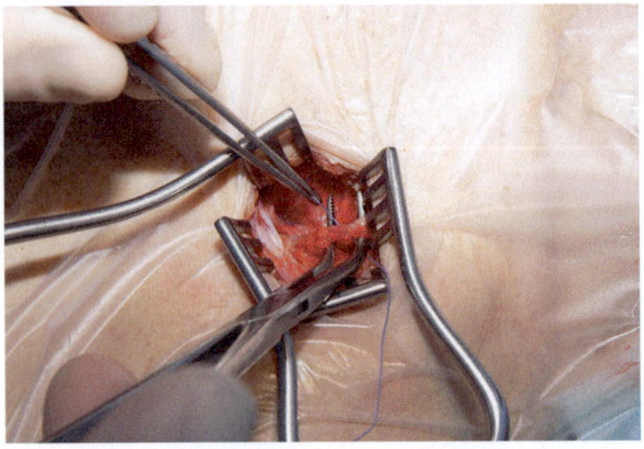

Fig. 10.9 Looping of the cephalic vein caudally and cranially. (© R. Hennes; all rights reserved)

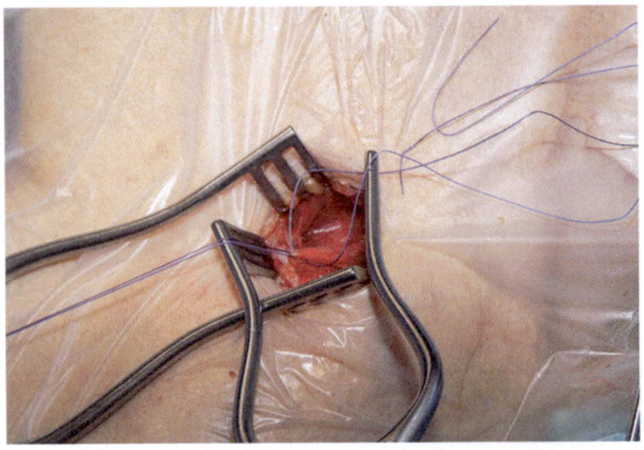

Fig. 10.10 Looping of the cephalic vein caudally and cranially. (© R. Hennes; all rights reserved)

10.4 Positioning the Port Catheter Tip

Ideally, the tip of the port catheter should be positioned just before the atrium. In a study, Baskin demonstrated that the optimal position is approximately 1–2 vertebral bodies below the bifurcation of the main bronchus (Baskin et al. 2008). This can be readily visualized intraoperatively using fluoroscopy. Because the port catheter is radiopaque, its course and position can be clearly delineated, enabling precise placement of the catheter tip at the atrial level (Fig. 10.14).

▶ **Practical Tip** In rare cases, the catheter may appear to be correctly positioned in the anteroposterior projection during image intensifier control, but is actually located in the internal mammary vein or the azygos vein. These positions can mimic the correct radiographic appearance. To prevent such malpositioning, a brief period of continuous intraoperative fluoroscopy can be performed to observe catheter tip movement, which serves as a reliable indicator of correct atrial placement (see Chap. 16).

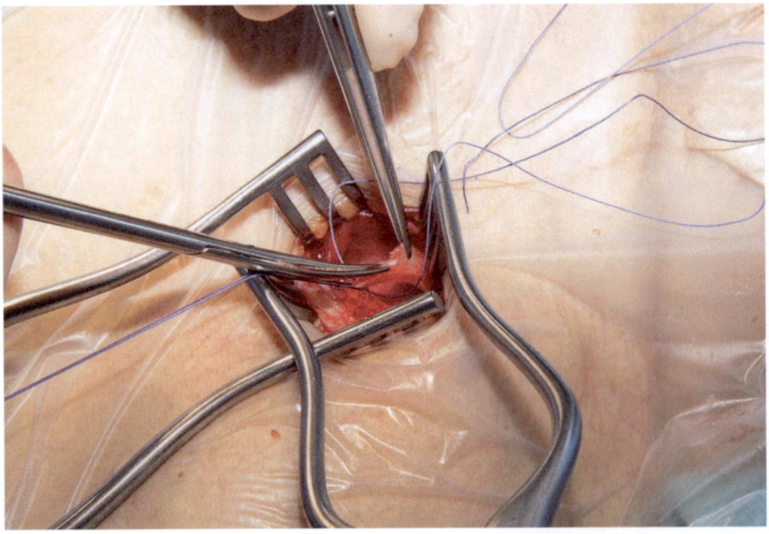

Fig. 10.11 Venotomy of the cephalic vein. (© R. Hennes; all rights reserved)

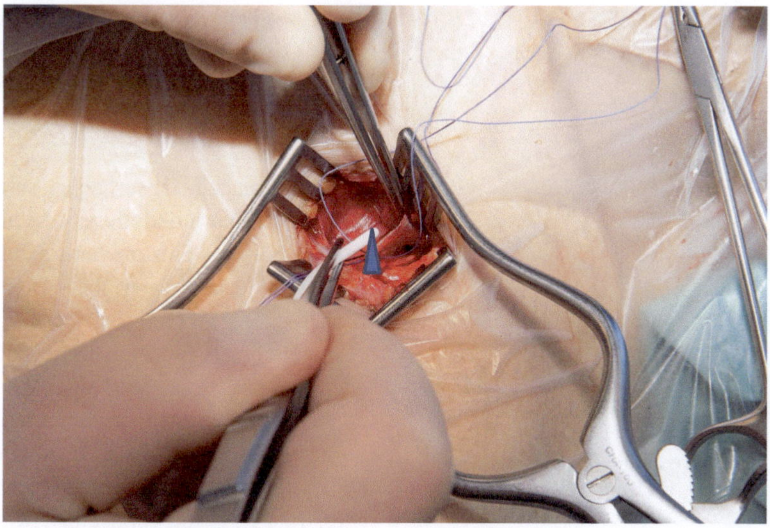

Fig. 10.12 With the left hand, forceps are used to keep the lumen of the cephalic vein open while the port catheter (6.6 F) is inserted. Note the tapered tip of the catheter, marked by the blue arrow. (© R. Hennes; all rights reserved)

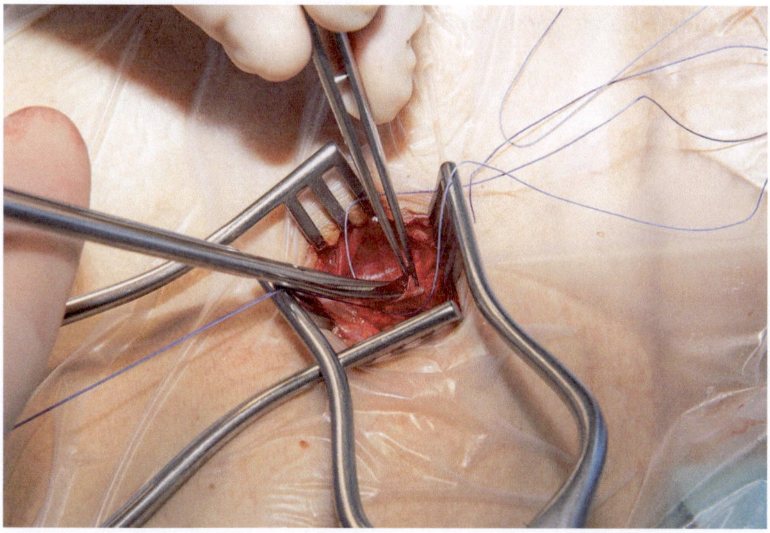

Fig. 10.13 After venotomy: Inserting the scissors into the lumen of the vein and spreading it open. (© R. Hennes; all rights reserved)

Intraoperative fluoroscopy is the safest and simplest method Alternatively ECG guidance may be used, which relies on ECG monitoring via the port catheter. For this the catheter is advanced until the P wave amplitude is maximized and withdrawn until the P wave returns to normal. When comparing these two methods, intraoperative fluoroscopy using an image intensifier remains the most reliable approach and should always be available, even when ECG guidance is used. This is particularly important in repeat procedures, where vascular anomalies or other factors may lead to catheter malposition, such as migration into the jugular vein (catheter kinking), azygos vein, internal mammary vein, or other unintended pathways—all of which

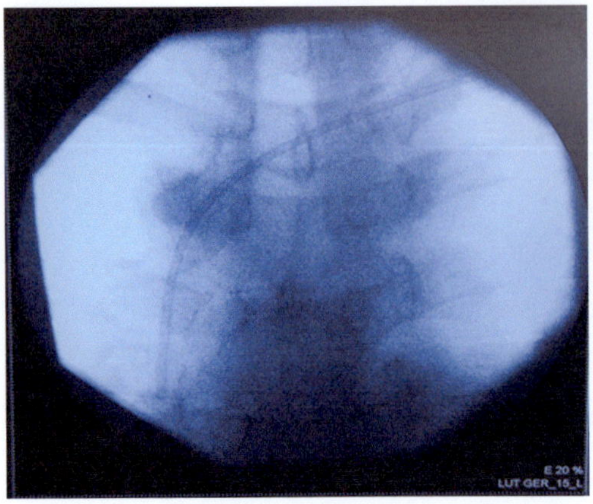

Fig. 10.14 Intraoperative radiographic control with a mobile image intensifier, showing correct positioning of the catheter tip approximately one vertebral body below the carina. (© R. Hennes; all rights reserved)

require intraoperative correction. The main limitation of the ECG method is its lack of signal in such cases, preventing accurate confirmation of atrial positioning.

10.5 Fixation and Connection of the Port Catheter to the Port Chamber and Creation of the Port Pocket

The pre-placed absorbable sutures on the cephalic vein are tied, thereby securing the catheter to the vein. This prevents subsequent retraction of the catheter into the subcutaneous tissue (Fig. 10.15).

After correct placement, the catheter is shortened and connected to the port chamber via the connector. This step is particularly critical for high-pressure ports, as it ensures the catheter's ability to withstand elevated injection pressures (Fig. 10.16). If the connector—whether inserted or screwed into the port chamber depending on the manufacturer—is not properly secured, the catheter may detach from the port chamber, especially during contrast administration or under infusion pump pressure, leading to extravasation. A thorough understanding of the

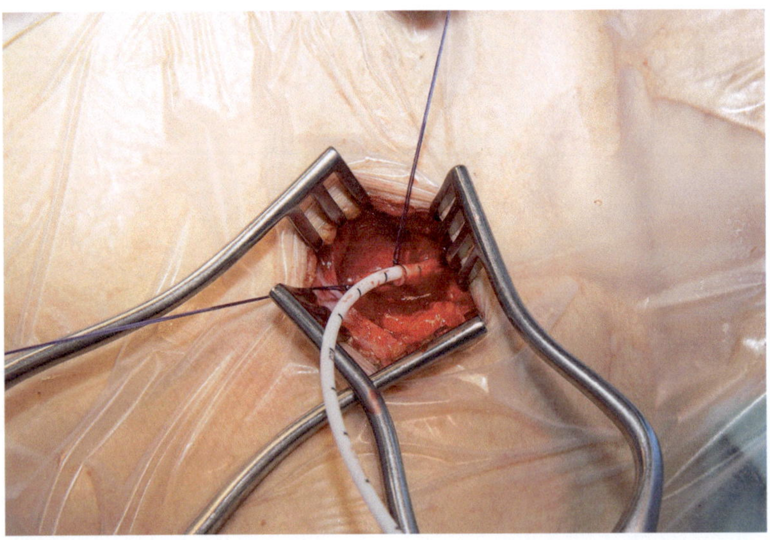

Fig. 10.15 After positioning the port catheter, ligation is performed caudally and cranially to secure the port catheter to the vein. (© R. Hennes; all rights reserved)

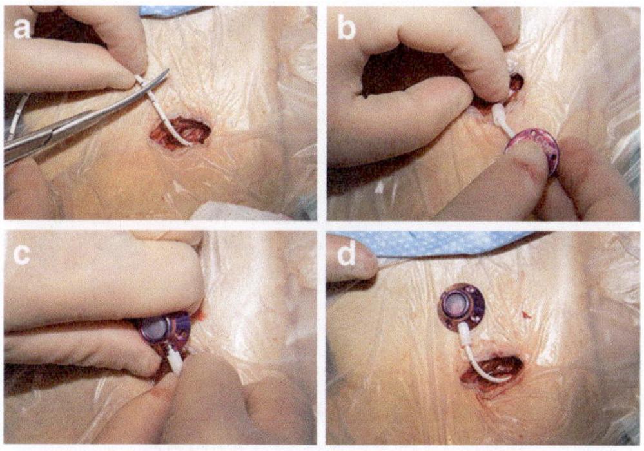

Fig. 10.16 a–d Shortening the port catheter and connecting it to the port chamber. It is crucial to establish a correct connection via the connector sleeve to the port chamber. (© R. Hennes; all rights reserved)

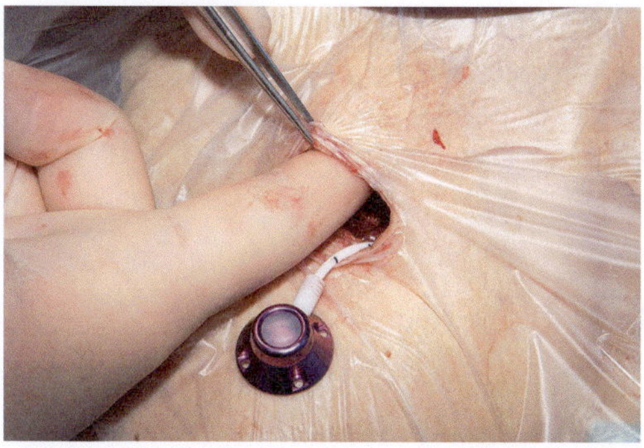

Fig. 10.17 Blunt dissection of the port pocket

assembly process, including correct attachment of the port catheter to the port chamber and proper connection of the connector sleeve, is therefore essential.

For training and education of residents, practicing the correct assembly and connection of the port chamber, connector unit, and port catheter as a "dry run" has proven effective.

After proper connection, the port chamber is placed on the pectoralis muscle approximately 2 cm medial to the incision line. Care should be taken not to create an unnecessarily large port pocket, as this can lead to additional trauma, bleeding, and hematoma formation. The port pocket should be expanded only as much as necessary to allow the port chamber to rest freely without tension, enabling its secure fixation to the pectoral fascia with at least two sutures (Figs. 10.17 and 10.18).

Fixation of the Port Chamber in Obese Patients

In our experience, fixation of the port chamber within adipose tissue in obese patients has not proven effective. While it is technically feasible, in very obese patients—who may have a subcutaneous tissue thickness of more than 8 cm in the pectoral region—placement in the fat tissue makes subsequent puncture and use of the port catheter extremely difficult, often resulting in failed punctures and additional trauma to the patient. We therefore always recommend fixation on the fascia of the pectoralis muscle.

> **Practical Tip** In very obese patients with a pronounced subcutaneous fat layer, we recommend reducing the subcutaneous fat above the port chamber to ensure easy and safe access to the port chamber later on.

In obese patients, puncturing the port chamber can be challenging, even when a larger

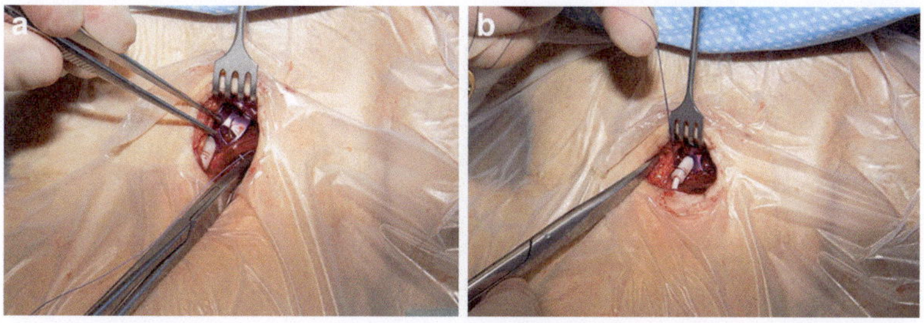

Fig. 10.18 a, b Suturing the port chamber to the pectoralis muscle with two fixation sutures. (© R. Hennes; all rights reserved)

chamber is used. To facilitate access, the overlying adipose tissue can be carefully reduced, which significantly improves palpation of the port chamber (Fig. 10.19). Any indentation over the port chamber caused by the procedure will remodel during the course of therapy. Thus, there is no lasting cosmetic issue. This approach effectively prevents failed punctures and reduces patient trauma from multiple needle sticks.

Another essential aspect of port implantation is securing the port chamber with fixation sutures, a step we strongly recommend. At least two sutures should be placed to anchor the chamber firmly (Fig. 10.18). At the Port Center of Heidelberg University Hospital, absorbable suture material is routinely used, as fibrous ingrowth and scarring around the port chamber typically occur within three to four weeks. This natural fixation maintains the port's position once the suture has dissolved and, unlike non-absorbable materials, prevents persistent nerve irritation resulting from contact or entrapment in the muscle layer. After the port chamber is secured, care must be taken to ensure that the catheter is not kinked and follows a gentle, semicircular course without tension or pressure on the deltoid muscle (Fig. 10.20).

10.6 Wound Closure and Functional Testing

The wound cavity is then irrigated and checked for hemostasis. For wound closure, we prefer a single- or double-layer subcutaneous suture (depending on the thickness of the subcutaneous fat tissue) to ensure secure closure of the subcutaneous spaces and to prevent hematoma formation. At the end of the procedure, the functionality of the port catheter must be checked (Fig. 10.21).

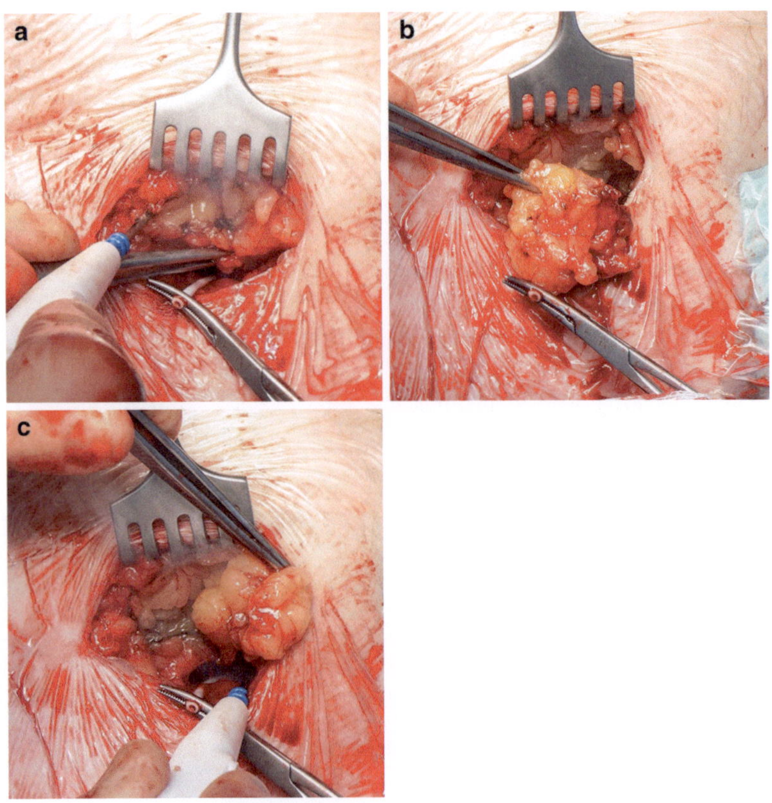

Fig. 10.19 **a–c** Reduction of subcutaneous fat tissue

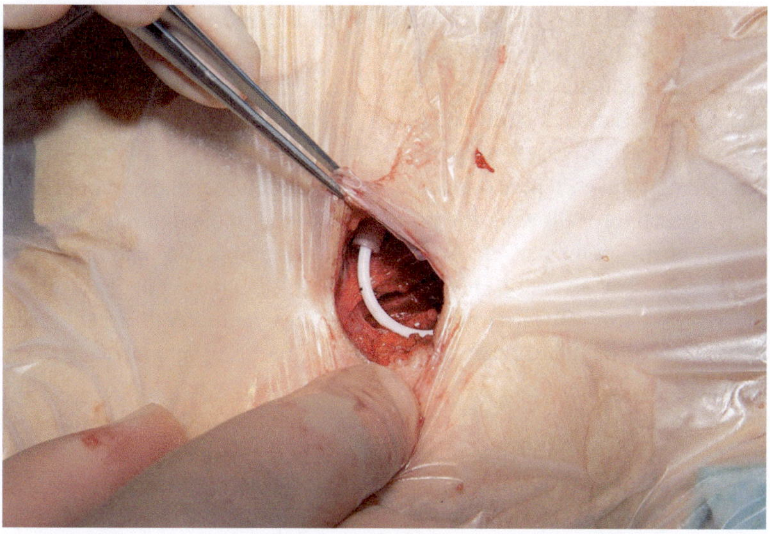

Fig. 10.20 After suturing the port chamber, care must be taken to ensure that the port catheter does not kink and enters the cephalic vein in a smooth curve. (© R. Hennes; all rights reserved)

In the present case, a port access needle was placed intraoperatively. It is crucial to verify that the port catheter allows free blood aspiration and can be flushed without resistance. If these functions are impaired, the position of the catheter tip must be re-evaluated, and, if necessary, intraoperative contrast administration should be performed to visualize the outflow.

For several years, skin closure has been performed exclusively with absorbable sutures. These dissolve after approximately 50 days according to the manufacturer. Clinical experience has shown that the immediate initiation of chemotherapy can adversely affect wound healing at the surgical site. When non-absorbable sutures were used and removed after 14 days,

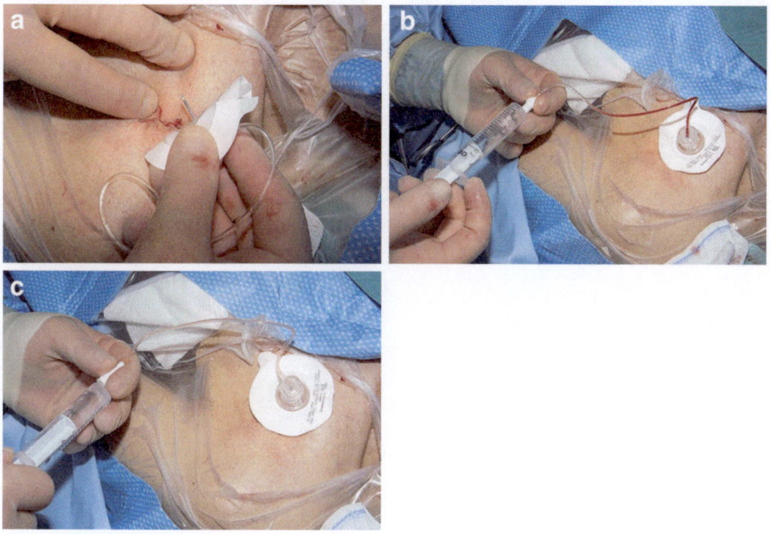

Fig. 10.21a–c Functional testing of the port catheter by aspiration (© R. Hennes; all rights reserved)

wound dehiscence and delayed healing were occasionally observed. This issue has been completely avoided through the routine use of absorbable sutures for wound closure in port implantation procedures. In cases requiring immediate chemotherapy, a port access needle can be placed intraoperatively, allowing the port to be used without any waiting period. At the Port Center of Heidelberg University Hospital, direct postoperative port use via intraoperative needle placement has been standard practice for the past ten years (Fig. 10.21).

The standard technique for port catheter implantation via venous cutdown of the cephalic vein, as performed at the Department of Surgery, Heidelberg University Hospital, is illustrated schematically in its essential steps in Fig. 10.22. The procedure can also be viewed as a video (see Fig. 10.23).

10.7 Impact of Proper Application of the Venous Cutdown Technique on Quality of Life

The quality of life of patients with implanted ports largely depends on both the proper execution of the implantation technique and the selection of appropriate materials. These factors are critical for ensuring patient comfort, ease of port handling, and overall acceptance of the device. Since the port chamber and catheter constitute a foreign body, they should be implanted in a manner that allows the port to be easily palpable, readily accessible for puncture, and securely stabilized during access, while minimizing patient discomfort. The patient's physical condition poses an additional challenge; in cases of severe obesity or cachexia, the surgical

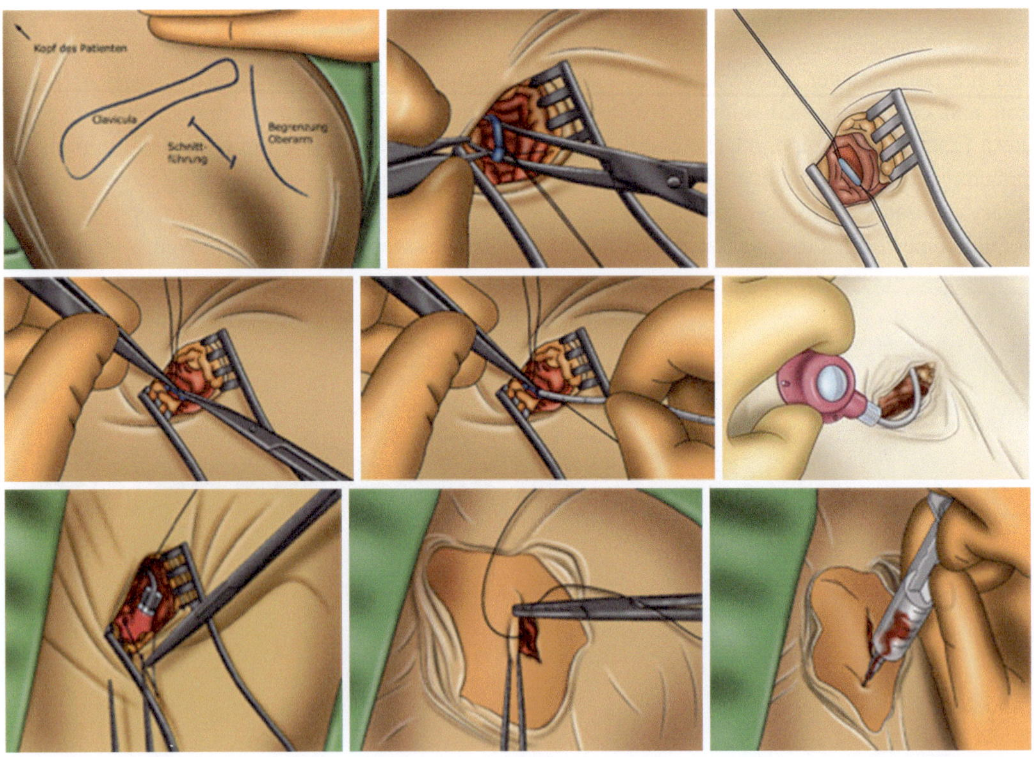

Fig. 10.22 Schematic representation of the standard technique via venous cutdown for port catheter implantation (Source Xope © Deutscher Ärzte-Verlag; all rights reserved)

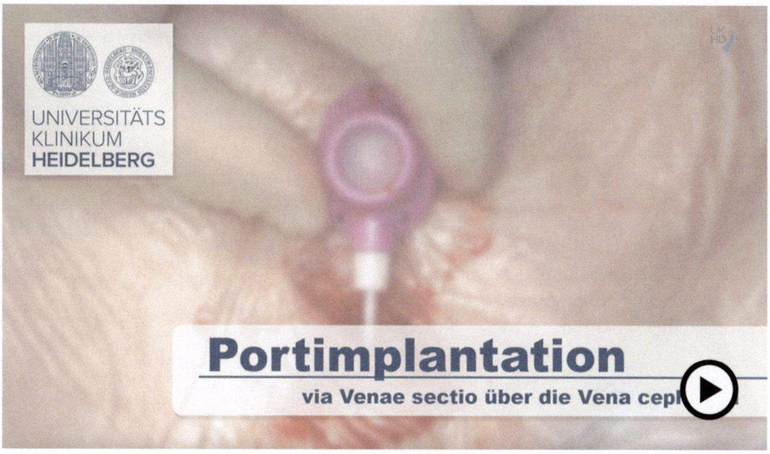

Fig. 10.23 Port implantation via venous cutdown of the cephalic vein. To play this video, please use the SN More Media app and scan the following URL: ▸ https://doi.org/10.1007/000-hgk

approach must be tailored to the individual anatomy and clinical circumstances.

Using the cephalic vein cutdown technique, the port can be positioned laterally enough to avoid extending into the décolleté while remaining outside the range of shoulder movement. When correctly placed and securely fixed, this positioning enables patients to engage in normal sporting and leisure activities without restriction. Careful preoperative planning, particularly regarding optimal incision placement, is essential for achieving a favorable cosmetic outcome. In patients of normal weight or slender build, an incision of approximately 3 cm is sufficient for port implantation via the cephalic vein in the deltopectoral groove. In obese patients, an incision extended to 4–5 cm is typically adequate to ensure proper implantation. When an intradermal absorbable suture technique with buried knots is used, patients may shower as early as the following day; swimming and bathing are generally permitted after ten days, provided wound healing is complete.

In the early postoperative period, patients often report a sensation of pressure, which is primarily related to the awareness of the implanted foreign body. Some also experience discomfort when wearing a seatbelt due to localized pressure over the port site. This can be easily alleviated by placing a small foam pad or cushion between the seatbelt and the port area, effectively reducing the sensation of pressure.

Many patients report dissatisfaction with a port catheter when they associate it with disease-related stigma and view its removal as a marker of "cure." In this context, it is the responsibility of the surgeon, nursing staff, and all involved colleagues to provide thorough patient education, ensuring that patients do not request premature port removal but instead understand that the indication for explantation should be determined by the responsible treating physician, based on clinical judgment and the overall course of treatment.

Drawing on the experience of more than 40,000 patients treated at the Port Center of Heidelberg University Hospital, port implantation via cephalic vein cutdown with placement of the port chamber on the chest wall medial to the deltopectoral groove has demonstrated excellent patient acceptance and provides maximal freedom of movement and quality of life. Furthermore, the risk of both intraoperative and postoperative complications associated with this technique is very low, particularly when compared with alternative central venous access devices. (see Chap. 16).

References

Baskin KM, Jimenez RM, Cahill AM, Jawad AF, Towbin RB (2008) Cavoatrial junction and central venous anatomy: implications for central venous access tip position. J Vasc Interv Radiol 19(3):359–365. https://doi.org/10.1016/j.jvir.2007.09.005. PMID: 18295694

Hennes R, Hofmann H (2016) Ports. Springer. ISBN 978-3-662-43640-0

Hüttner et al (2019) Primary open versus closed implantation strategy for totally implantable venous access ports. Ann Surg

Knebel P, Lopez-Benitez R, Fischer L et al (2011) Insertion of totally implantable venous access devices: an expertise-based, randomized, controlled trial (NCT00600444). Ann Surg 253:1111–1117

Puncture of the Subclavian Vein and the Jugular Vein

11

De-Hua Chang

▶ In addition to the traditional open surgical port placement, radiological interventional implantation techniques have become increasingly widespread over time (Funaki B et al. 1997; Shetty PC et al. 1997). Unlike the cut-down technique, in which the cephalic or jugular vein is typically exposed, these methods involve percutaneous puncture of the target vein—primarily the subclavian or internal jugular vein—either under ultrasound guidance or as a so-called blind puncture using anatomical landmarks. The catheter is then inserted using the Seldinger technique. This eliminates the need for vessel looping, venotomy, and ligation. Both the implantation method and the choice of venous access route carry distinct advantages and disadvantages. The following section provides a detailed description of the various clinically established approaches.

11.1 Introduction

Various methods and access routes are available for initial venous puncture during port catheter placement. Puncture can either be performed under ultrasound guidance or solely based on anatomical landmarks. The most common access routes are the internal jugular vein on the lateral side of the neck and the subclavian vein beneath the clavicle.

The theoretical advantage of the internal jugular vein approach lies in its straighter catheter course, which minimizes the risk of venous wall irritation or thrombosis caused by a tip positioned adjacent to the vessel wall. Additional benefits include easy external access and better management of serious complications, such as bleeding from inadvertent arterial puncture. Furthermore, the risk of pneumothorax is minimized by the peripheral puncture at the neck. In experienced hands, these complications are exceedingly rare and thus negligible in clinical practice. Due to heterogeneous data, a Cochrane analysis was unable to provide a definitive assessment regarding the preferred access route when considering complication rates and catheter function duration (Ge X et al. 2012). In addition to technical success rates, complication rates, and catheter longevity, anatomical conditions, surgicalrefi expertise, and patient preference are increasingly important factors selecting the access route.

(Hind D et al. 2003; Brass et al. 2015). Ultrasound-guided puncture has proven especially effective in obese patients with deep-seated veins or patients with congenitally narrow veins.

D.-H. Chang (✉)
Radiologie und Nuklearmedizin, Kantonsspital Luzern, Luzern, Switzerland
e-mail: de-hua.chang@luks.ch

R. Hennes (ed.), *Port Surgery*, https://doi.org/10.1007/978-3-662-70624-4_11

Various manufacturers offer specialized port sets for implantation using the Seldinger technique. These include a so-called peel-away introducer for catheter placement. Stiffer guidewires facilitate sheath placement, while puncture needles with echogenic tips are designed to enhance ultrasound visibility.

11.2 Planning the Sonographic Puncture

Subclavian Vein

The choice of side for subclavian vein port implantation depends on the underlying disease and, in cases of malignancy involving the thoracic inlet or neck, should be performed on the unaffected side. In the absence of such involvement, left-sided port placement is generally preferred for right-handed surgeons. With few exceptions (e.g., in anxious patients), the procedure is performed under local anesthesia. First, ultrasound is used to evaluate the patency of the subclavian vein. The area is then prepared in a sterile fashion, ensuring an adequately wide operative field that extends laterally to the level of the anterior axillary line. The patient's head is turned to the side opposite the implantation, and the sterile drape is tented over a frame to allow free breathing (Fig. 11.1). The surgeon is situated next to the patient's chest.

Internal Jugular Vein

Port placement via the internal jugular vein is preferred on the right side due to the shorter intravascular course of the catheter relative to the superior vena cava. The procedure is conducted similar to subclavian vein puncutre under local anasthesia, initially confirming vein patency via ultrasound. The sterile field should extend from the lateral side of the neck to 5 cm caudal to the clavicle (at the level of the intended port chamber implantation). The patient's head is turned to the side opposite the implantation. For the puncture, the surgeon stands at the head of the patient.

11.3 Implantation Procedure

V. subclavia

In principle, the ultrasound probe may be oriented either longitudinally or transversely to the subclavian vein. For anatomical reasons, a longitudinal alignment is recommended. To achieve this, the probe is positioned parallel and just inferior to the clavicle and then slowly advanced caudally until the subclavian vein comes into view. The transducer should rest orthogonally on the skin without tilting. By gently rotating the probe clockwise or counterclockwise, the V. subclavia may be visualized in a straight line along its course (Fig. 11.2). It is important to identify the spatial relationship to the subclavian artery a few centimeters more cranially to avoid inadvertent arterial puncture. Before venipuncture, ultrasound-guided local anesthetic is administered along the planned access route from the skin to just superficial to the vein, and additional local anesthesia is infiltrated into the skin and subcutaneous tissue over the intended incision and port chamber pocket.

> **Practical Tip** In case of very narrow veins, a Valsalva maneuver can dilate the vessels and facilitate puncture. Care should be taken to maintain intrathoracic pressure until the guidewire has been inserted. Premature exhalation may cause the vein to collapse and result in needle displacement, so the breathing maneuver should be practiced with the patient in advance.
>
> As the caliber of the V. subclavia increases along its course, some surgeons prefer to puncture the vein in the medial segment below the clavicle. However, puncture of the V. subclavia in the lateral segment offers some advantages: firstly, needle visualization below the clavicle is limited or absent due to acoustic shadowing, increasing the risk of accidental deep puncture and subsequent pneumothorax. Secondly, mechanical catheter complications, such as the so-called pinch-off syndrome—extravasal compression

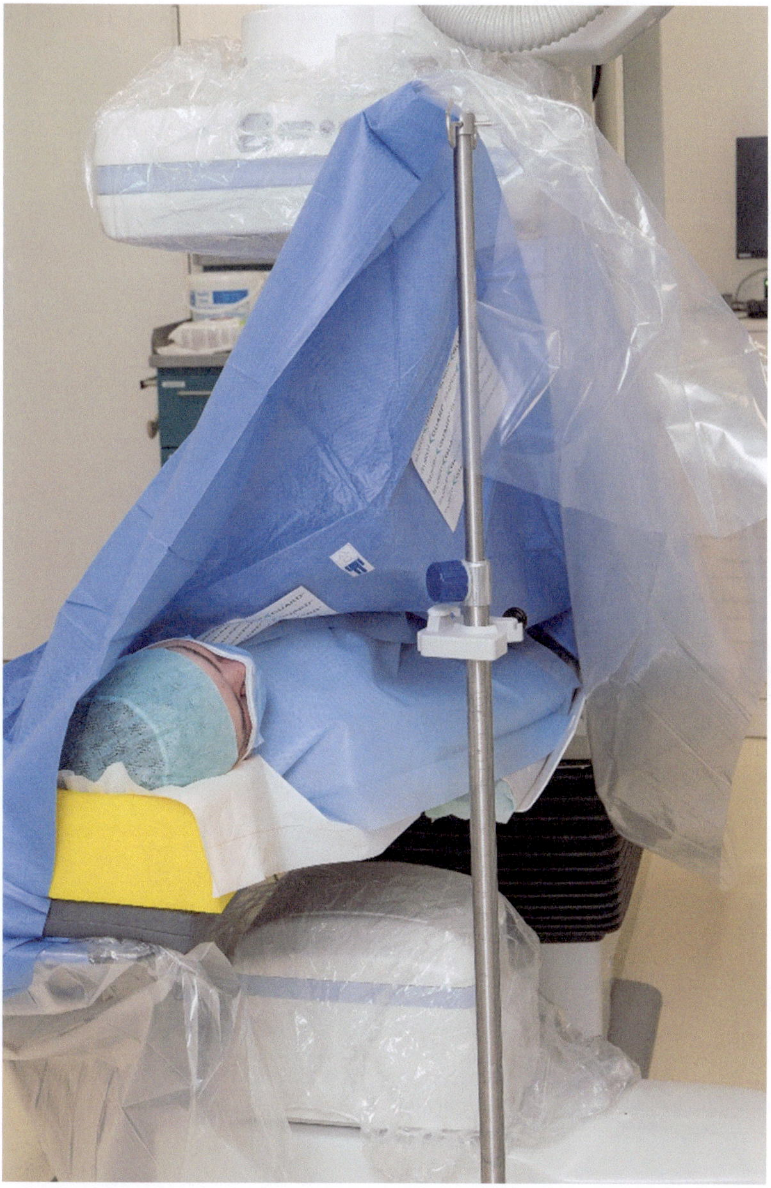

Fig. 11.1 Positioning of the patient for ultrasound-guided puncture of the left subclavian vein

of the catheter between the clavicle and first rib with risk of catheter fracture—are avoided.

After a small skin incision, the anterior wall of the V. subclavia is punctured using a 10-ml locking syringe. Successful aspiration of blood confirms correct intravascular placement. We recommend advancing the guidewire under fluoroscopic guidance. The wire should be positioned in the right atrium or the right V. cava inferior. If this cannot be confirmed, a second projection in another plane should be obtained to exclude malposition of the wire in a side branch (V. thoracica interna, V. azygos, etc.). After confirming correct wire placement, the peel-away sheath is introduced using the Seldinger technique. The port catheter is clamped distally

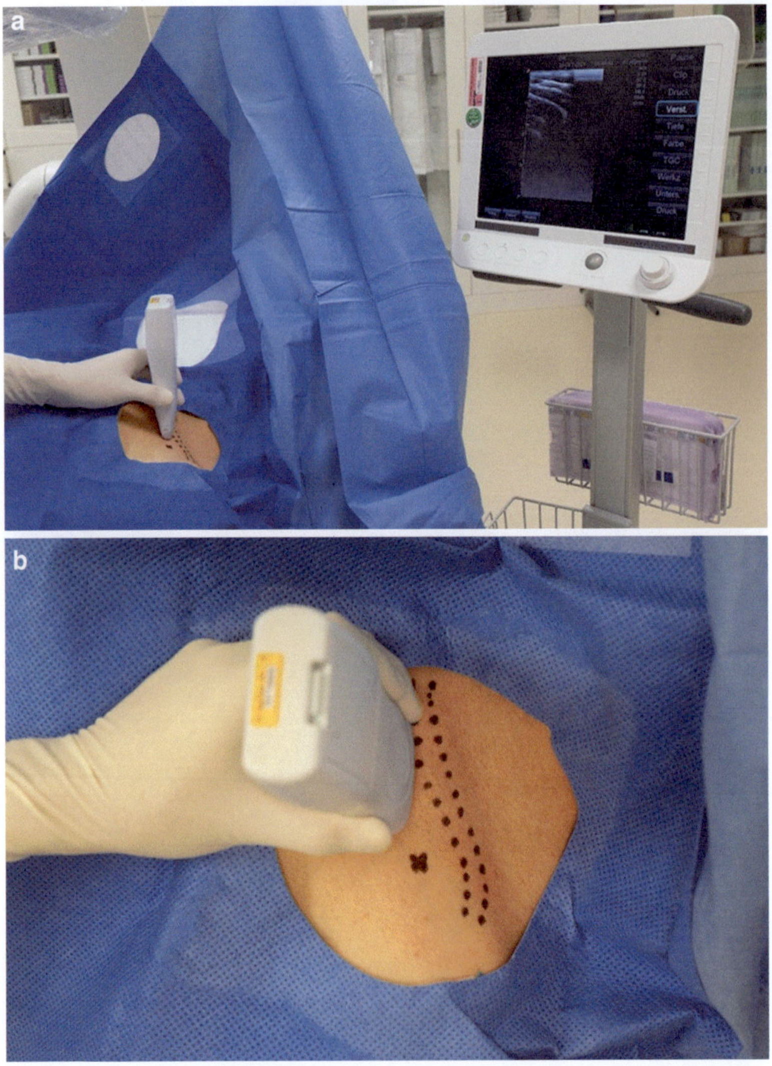

Fig. 11.2 Demonstration of ultrasound probe positioning for puncture of the left V. subclavia. Dashed line = course of the clavicle; cross = puncture site of the needle

and inserted into the sheath. The catheter tip should initially be placed in the right atrium and only withdrawn to the cavoatrial junction after removal of the sheath. (Advancing the catheter after sheath removal is significantly more difficult due to frictional resistance.)

Next, a 3–4 cm transverse skin incision is made, followed by creation of a subcutaneous pocket via blunt dissection. The pocket for the port chamber should be positioned a few centimeters below the skin incision to minimize wound healing complications from subsequent needle punctures during port use. Two absorbable sutures are preplaced on the fascia of the M. pectoralis to secure the port chamber at the end of the procedure.

If the catheter has a longer subcutaneous course, a tunneling rod can be used to guide the catheter. The rod is advanced from the cutaneous puncture site toward the port pocket. The catheter is attached to the end of the rod and pulled through the subcutaneous tissue. It is then trimmed to the appropriate length and connected to the port chamber.

The port catheter is checked for leaks and, if necessary, sealed with heparin. The chamber is fixed to the fascia with the preplaced sutures, and the wound is closed.

After implantation, a chest X-ray is performed to rule out pneumothorax.

V. jugularis interna
In contrast to the subclavian vein, for which an in-plane ultrasound approach is preferred, internal jugular vein puncture is best performed using an out-of-plane probe orientation. The transducer is placed on the lateral neck at the level of the cricoid, and the V. jugularis and A. carotis are identified. During advancement, the needle tip is continuously tracked by moving the ultrasound probe caudally. Local anesthesia should cover the access route as well as the subcutaneous course of the catheter along the lateral neck, over the clavicle, and into the pectoral port pocket.

▶ **Practical Tip** The exact position of the needle tip can often be better confirmed using small, jerky in-and-out movements. If uncertainty persists, switching to the longitudinal (in-plane) view can be helpful. With slow needle advancement, anterior wall indentation just before venous entry is not uncommon.

The subsequent steps are the same as for catheter insertion via the V. subclavia. For subcutaneous tunneling of the catheter, use of the tunneling rod is necessary. Under fluoroscopy, in addition to confirming correct catheter position at the cavoatrial junction, particular attention should be paid to excluding kinking of the catheter at the vessel entry site.

Puncture Using Anatomical Landmarks
The success of landmark-guided puncture of the V. subclavia or V. jugularis depends on whether the target vein is in the expected position, is patent, and has sufficient caliber. It should be noted that ultrasound-guided puncture is safer and has a higher success rate. If an ultrasound device is not available, the following approach may be used.

V. subclavia
After local anesthesia and a small skin incision, the needle is inserted 1–2 cm below the clavicle at the level of the midclavicular line. The cannula is then advanced under aspiration parallel to the skin, directly beneath the clavicle, toward the jugular notch. After successful blood aspiration, the procedure continues as described for ultrasound-guided puncture (see Sect. 11.3).

V. jugularis interna
First, the A. carotis is identified by palpation. After local anesthesia and a small skin incision, the puncture needle is inserted at the level of the palpable pulse. The direction of puncture is strictly lateral to avoid inadvertent arterial puncture. After blood aspiration, the procedure continues as described for ultrasound-guided puncture (see Sect. 11.3).

References

Brass P, Hellmich M, Kolodziej L, Schick G, Smith AF (2015) Ultrasound guidance versus anatomical landmarks for internal jugular vein catheterization. Cochrane Database Syst Rev 9;1(1):CD006962. https://doi.org/10.1002/14651858.CD006962.pub2

Funaki B, Szymski GX, Hackworth CA, Rosenblum JD, Burke R, Chang T, Leef JA (1997) Radiologic placement of subcutaneous infusion chest ports for long-term central venous access. AJR Am J Roentgenol 169(5):1431–1434. https://doi.org/10.2214/ajr.169.5.9353475

Ge X, Cavallazzi R, Li C, Pan SM, Wang YW, Wang FL (2012) Central venous access sites for the prevention of venous thrombosis, stenosis and infection. Cochrane Database Syst Rev 14(3):CD004084. https://doi.org/10.1002/14651858.CD004084.pub3

Hind D, Calvert N, McWilliams R, Davidson A, Paisley S, Beverley C, Thomas S (2003) Ultrasonic locating devices for central venous cannulation: meta-analysis. BMJ 16;327(7411):361. https://doi.org/10.1136/bmj.327.7411.361

Shetty PC, Mody MK, Kastan DJ, Sharma RP, Burke MW, Venugopal C, Burke TH (1997) Outcome of 350 implanted chest ports placed by interventional radiologists. J Vasc Interv Radiol 8(6):991–995. https://doi.org/10.1016/s1051-0443(97)70699-7

Part IV

Implantation Techniques for Revision Procedures, Specialized Methods, and Port Explantation

Venous Section and Puncture in the Groin Area

12

Roland Hennes

Inserting ports or Hickman catheters via the groin is an alternative approach that we have successfully practiced at the Heidelberg Port Center for over 10 years (Hennes and Hofman 2016). One of the key aspects of postoperative care for ports and Hickman catheters is maintaining strict hygiene. The groin area, being in close proximity to the genital and anal regions, may be at higher risk for contamination due to increased microbial colonization. This raises various questions about how to safely place catheters in this region without increasing the risk of infection. Ports implanted via the groin can remain in the body for years.

12.1 Key Aspects and Fundamentals of Port and Hickman Catheter Implantation via the Groin

The goal of placing a port or Hickman catheter should always be to provide a long-term (years) solution. This applies equally to catheters placed via the groin. At the same time, it is essential to ensure that the care and use of the catheters can be performed without complications.

In this chapter, we focus primarily on the venous cutdown technique. Puncture of the groin vessels is routinely and safely performed under ultrasound guidance in anesthesia and can be applied in the same way for port and Hickman catheters. However, this technique also requires tunneling and placement of the port chamber. This necessitates an extended incision in the groin to safely and easily position the catheter, as well as an additional incision on the lateral thigh over the tensor fasciae latae muscle.

If no superficial or easily accessible vein such as the great saphenous vein can be identified, we switch to a simple open puncture of the femoral vein.

Indications for Placement of a Port or Hickman Catheter via the Groin

- Bilateral thrombosis of the subclavian and jugular veins
- Superior vena cava syndrome
- Cardiac and thoracic surgery with complex anatomical conditions
- Other situations that make placement via the thorax impossible

R. Hennes (✉)
Klinik für Allgemein-, Viszeral- und Transplantationschirurgie, Universitätsklinikum Heidelberg, Heidelberg, Germany
e-mail: Roland.Hennes@med.uni-heidelberg.de

R. Hennes (ed.), *Port Surgery*, https://doi.org/10.1007/978-3-662-70624-4_12

12.2 Planning and Surgical Procedure

First, careful planning of the side to be operated on should be carried out.

Even in the groin area, factors such as thrombosis, vascular prostheses, and bypass circuits render placement via the groin impossible.

Therefore, preoperative assessment of venous outflow should always be performed.

This can be done using ultrasound or more advanced imaging techniques.

An image intensifier must be available for intraoperative catheter position control.

The tip of the port catheter should be placed only a few centimeters beyond the confluence of the iliac vessels into the inferior vena cava.

Catheter positioning at the level of the kidneys is strictly to be avoided, as catheter-associated thrombosis could compromise renal function. If adequate position control with the image intensifier is not possible due to an obese abdomen, venous outflow can be assessed using contrast agents. In the case of contrast agent allergy, the position of the catheter can be visualized by introducing a guidewire.

12.2.1 Surgical Steps

Step 1
After planning the incision for tunneling and placement of the port chamber (Fig. 12.1), a straight incision approximately 7 cm long is made below the inguinal ligament in the groin area. Ideally, the port chamber should be placed in the proximal, lateral thigh region over the tensor fasciae latae muscle. This provides a good support for the port chamber and facilitates puncture of the port chamber, even in obese patients.

Step 2
After incising the skin and subcutaneous tissue, self-retaining retractors are inserted (Fig. 12.2).

▶ **Practical Tip** When positioning the patient, ensure that the pelvis/lower abdomen does not lie over the operating table column, as this hinders position control with the image intensifier!

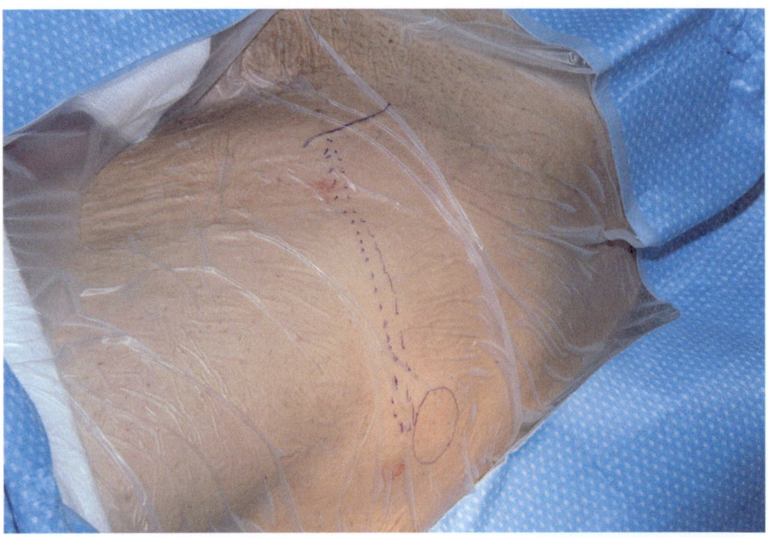

Fig. 12.1 Marking the incision in the left groin with planned tunneling and placement of the port chamber on the lateral side of the proximal thigh. (© R. Hennes; all rights reserved)

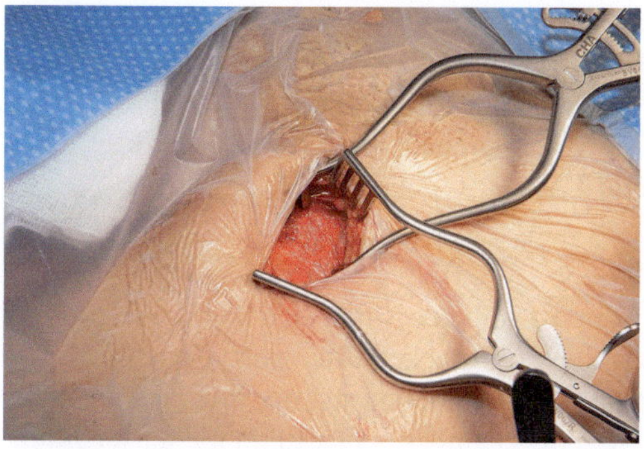

Fig. 12.2 Incision of the skin and subcutaneous tissue with insertion of self-retaining retractors.

Step 3

Identification of a superficial vein for subsequent port catheter implantation. As described, there are several options with additional venous tributaries, such as the great saphenous vein (Fig. 12.3).

Step 4

Looping the vein distally and cranially in preparation for the venous cutdown (Fig. 12.4).

Step 5

Perform the venous dissection to insert the port catheter and, if necessary, the guidewire. To do this, make an incision approximately one-third of the vein's diameter and immediately use scissors to gently widen the vein. This approach speeds up the insertion of the port catheter and is more effective than using the supplied vein hook ("shoe") as an intermediate step.

With good venous outflow the port catheter can be advanced directly into the inferior vena cava (Figs. 12.5 and 12.6).

> **Practical Tip** The port catheter should be positioned only a few centimeters beyond the confluence of the iliac vessels into the inferior vena cava! The port catheter should never be placed at the level of the kidneys, as catheter-associated thrombosis in this location can severely compromise renal function.

Step 6

Controlled advancement of the port catheter is performed under fluoroscopic guidance. As described above, contrast agents or a guidewire can be used to aid visualization (Figs. 12.7 and 12.8).

Step 7

Tie the pre-placed sutures to the vein and close distally. If the femoral vein is punctured, the Seldinger technique is used. Care must be

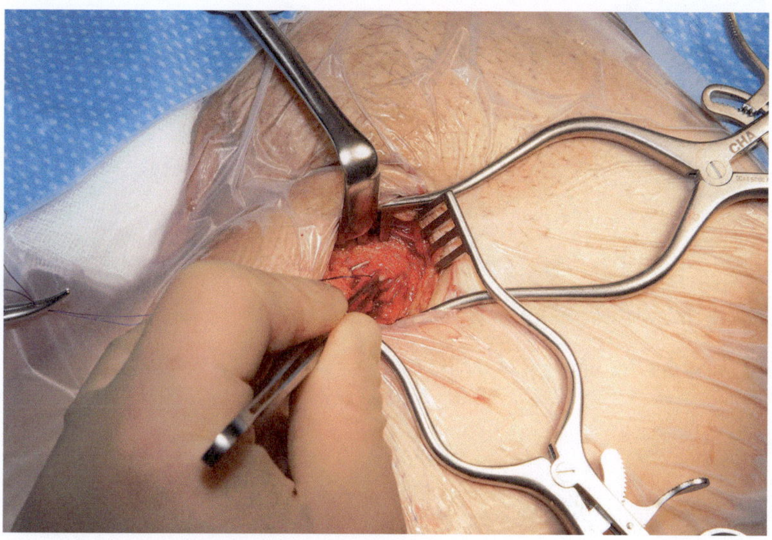

Fig. 12.3 Identification of the vein to be used for subsequent implantation.

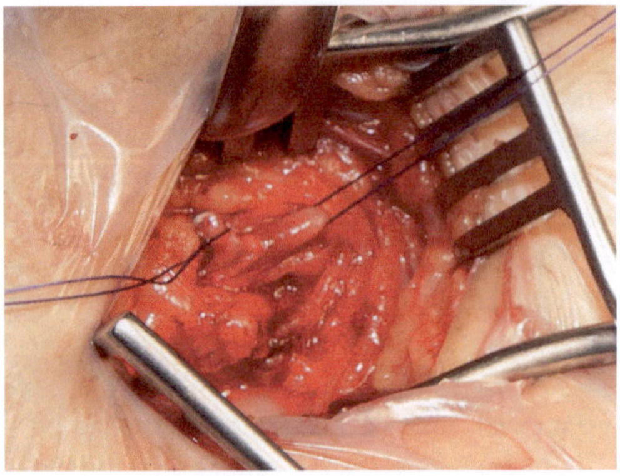

Fig. 12.4 Looping the vein cranially and distally. (© R. Hennes; all rights reserved)

taken to ensure that the catheter does not kink and is tunneled laterally in a smooth curve (Fig. 12.9).

Step 8

Make an incision over the proximal lateral aspect of the thigh, expose the tensor fasciae latae, and prepare the port pocket (Figs. 12.10 and 12.11).

Step 9

The port catheter is tunneled and passed through to the port pocket. The port catheter is then trimmed and connected to the port chamber. The port chamber is placed on the tensor fasciae latae and sutured in place (Figs. 12.12, 12.13, 12.14, 12.15, 12.16, 12.17, 12.18, and 12.19). It is essential to ensure that the port catheter does not kink.

Step 10

Closure of the skin incisions with an intracutaneous suture and functional testing of the port system by puncturing the port chamber, aspirating blood, flushing, and locking with saline (Fig. 12.20).

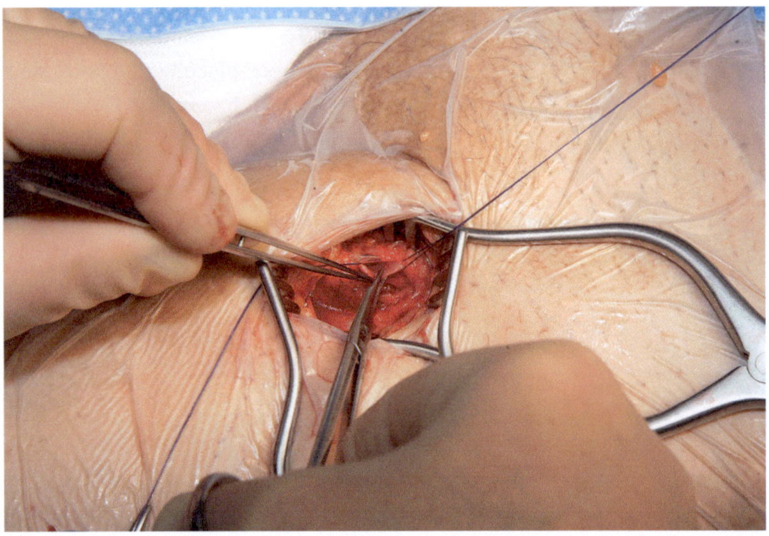

Fig. 12.5 Venous dissection for insertion of the port catheter and, if necessary, the guidewire. (© R. Hennes; all rights reserved)

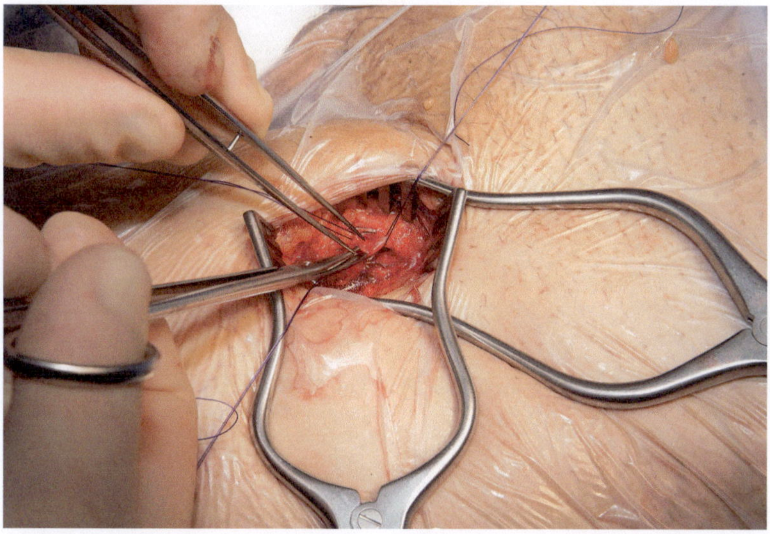

Fig. 12.6 After venous dissection, insert the scissors and spread the vein. (© R. Hennes; all rights reserved)

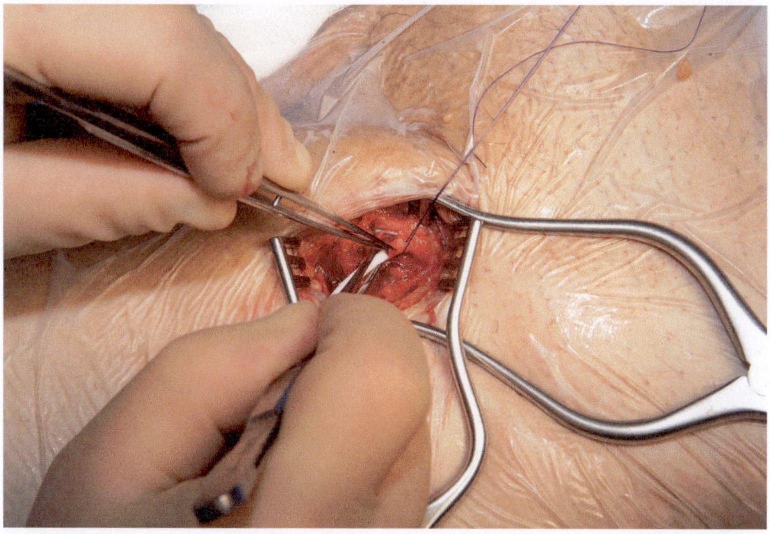

Fig. 12.7 Insertion of the port catheter, 6.6 F polyurethane, and advancement under fluoroscopic guidance. (© R. Hennes; all rights reserved)

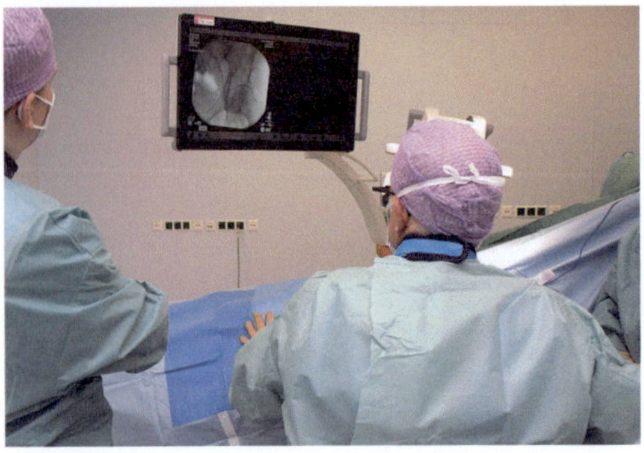

Fig. 12.8 Position check of the port catheter. (© R. Hennes; all rights reserved)

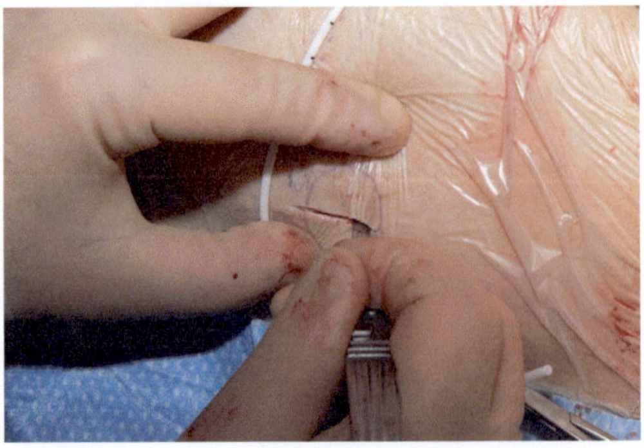

Fig. 12.10 Incision on the lateral aspect of the proximal thigh. (© R. Hennes; all rights reserved)

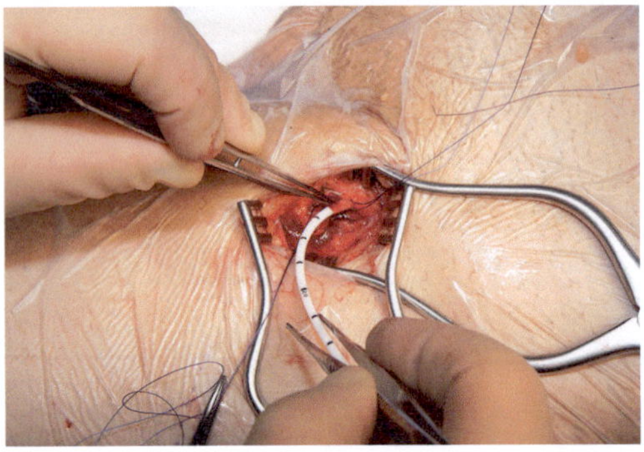

Fig. 12.9 The pre-placed sutures are tied to the superficial vein and closed distally. (© R. Hennes; all rights reserved)

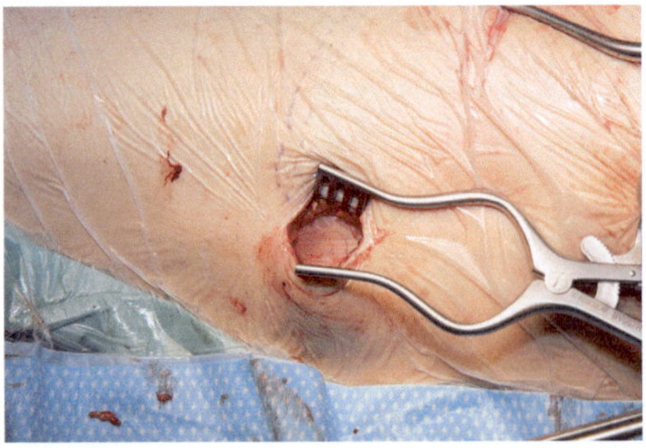

Fig. 12.11 Exposure of the tensor fasciae latae for placement of the port chamber. (© R. Hennes; all rights reserved)

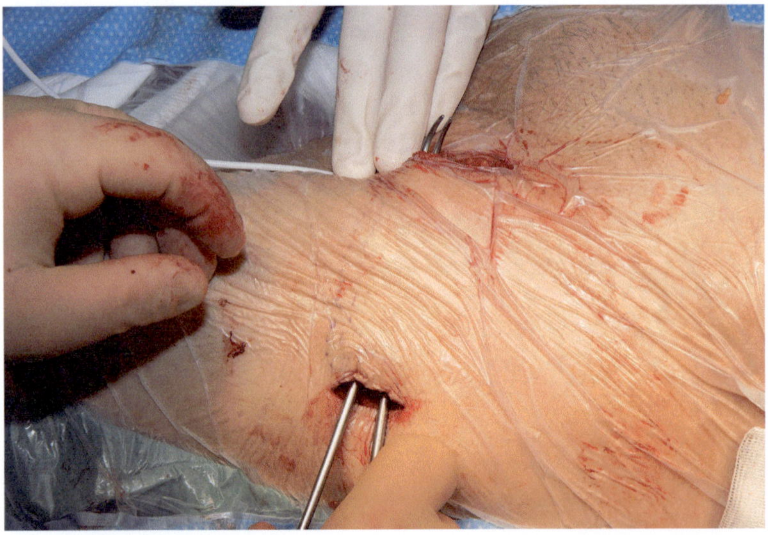

Fig. 12.12 Tunneling with the Overholt. (© R. Hennes; all rights reserved)

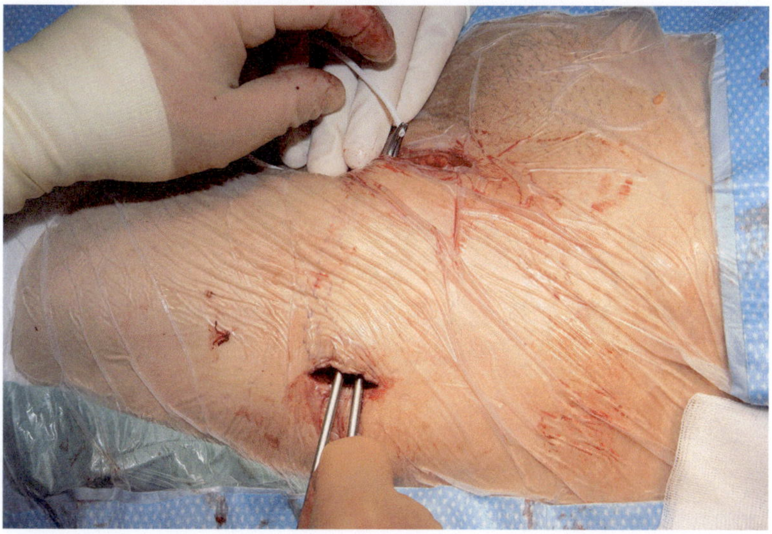

Fig. 12.13 Grasping the end of the port catheter and controlled passage into the port pocket. (© R. Hennes; all rights reserved)

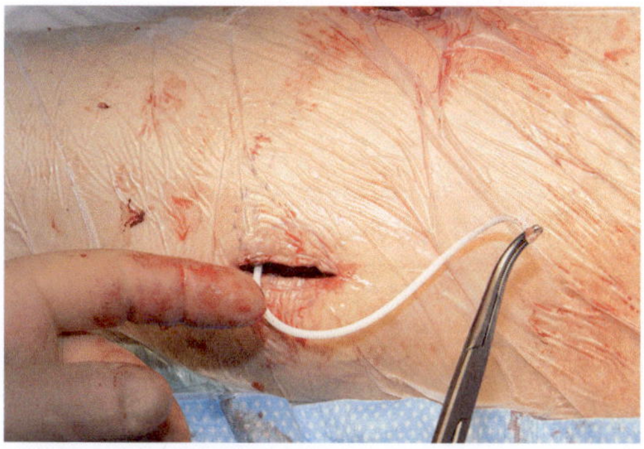

Fig. 12.14 Port catheter passed through, to be connected to the port chamber without kinking. (© R. Hennes; all rights reserved)

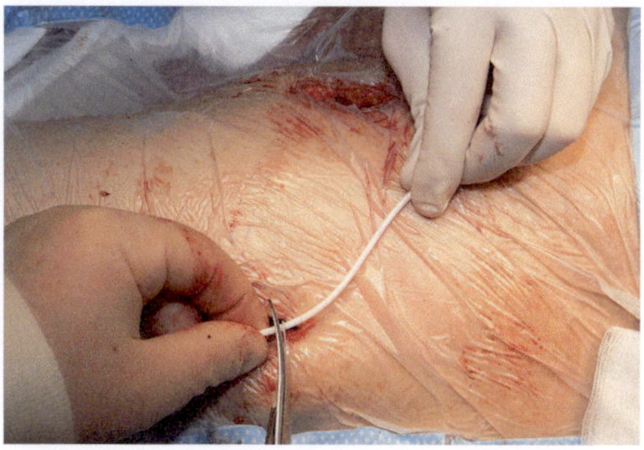

Fig. 12.15 Trimming the catheter. (© R. Hennes; all rights reserved)

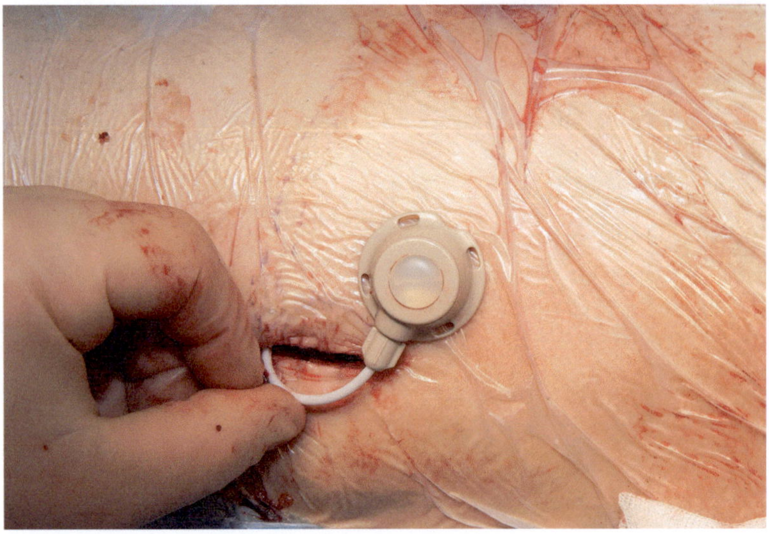

Fig. 12.16 Connection to the port chamber. (© R. Hennes; all rights reserved)

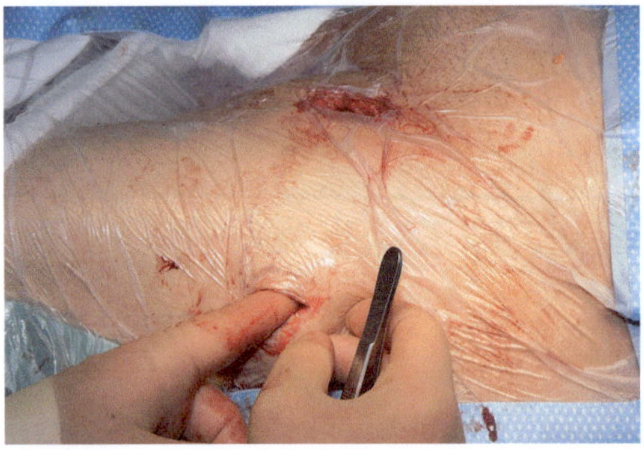

Fig. 12.17 Blunt dissection of the port pocket for placement of the port chamber. (© R. Hennes; all rights reserved)

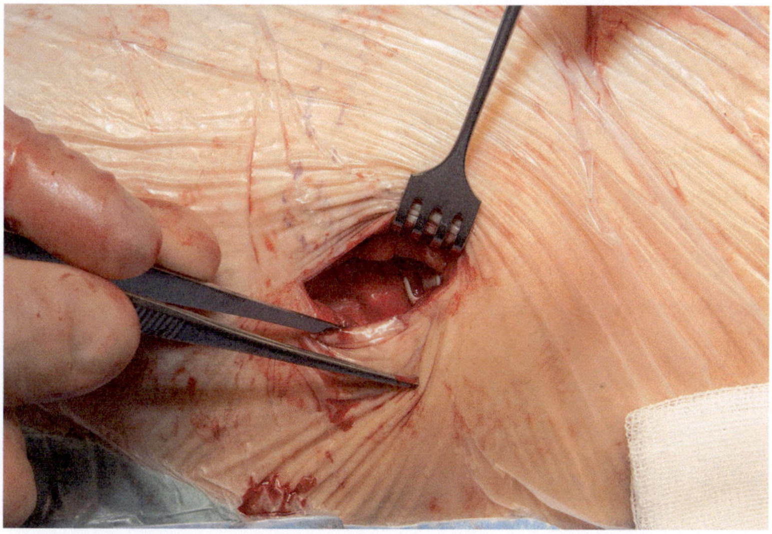

Fig. 12.18 Placement of the port chamber on the tensor fasciae latae. (© R. Hennes; all rights reserved)

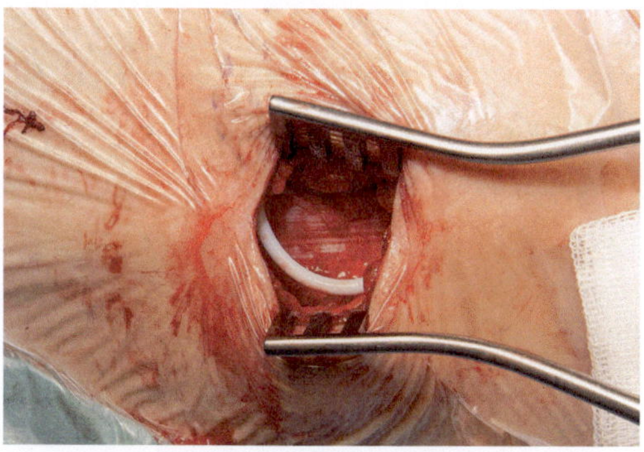

Fig. 12.19 Ensuring a smooth catheter course without kinking. (© R. Hennes; all rights reserved)

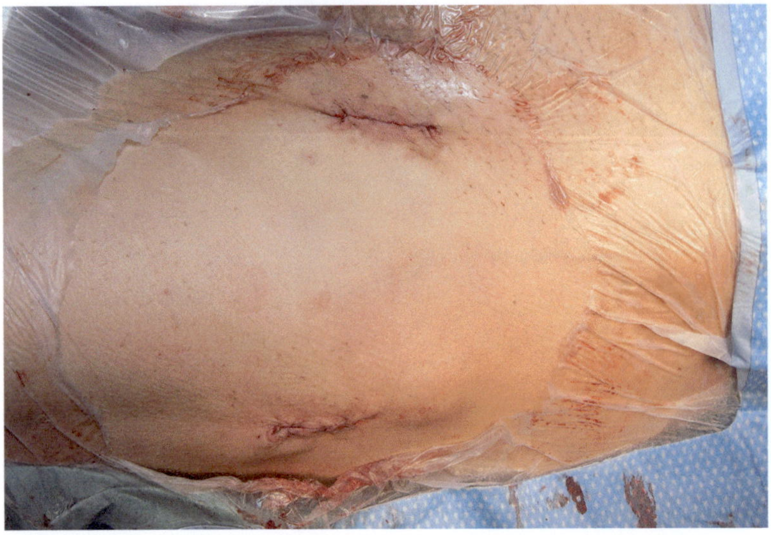

Fig. 12.20 Closure of both wounds with an intracutaneous suture. (© R. Hennes; all rights reserved)

Reference

Hennes R, Hofmann H (2016) Ports. Springer. ISBN 978-3-662-43640-0

Modified Seldinger Technique and Microsurgical Procedures for Port and Hickman Implantation

13

Roland Hennes

▶ A key challenge for surgeons during port implantation is the substantial variation in venous anatomy, with veins presenting a wide range of calibers. The ideally large-caliber cephalic vein- preferred for straightforward placement of the port catheter via venous cutdown- is not always available in the desired diameter. This is especially true in reoperations and revisions, where additional techniques are required to ensure safe and competent patient care. The modified Seldinger technique is one such method, providing versatile options for successful port implantation in nearly all clinical scenarios

A key challenge for surgeons during port implantation is the substantial variation in venous anatomy, with veins presenting a wide range of calibers. The ideally large-caliber cephalic vein—preferred for straightforward port catheter placement via venous cutdown—is not always available in the desired diameter. It is frequently observed that even during primary procedures, anatomical conditions, prior surgeries, and especially reoperations can result in alteredand unfavorable circumstances. Furthermore, oncological patients frequently exhibit reduced veinous caliber, in the sense of very narrow or even thrombosed vessels. For adults, a port catheter diameter of 6.6 to 8 French has proven effective for implantation. Since veins are highly distensible, there is some leeway in this regard. Ultimately, however, surgical feasibility reaches its limit when the target vein measures as little as 1 mm—or even 0.5 mm—in diameter. This is particularly true in reoperations, where the cephalic vein has already been "used up" by previous procedures and can often no longer be utilized. For instance, there may be partial thromboses or very small accompanying veins of the pectoralis muscle. In such cases, the modified Seldinger technique provides an excellent method to overcome these obstacles and effectively utilize otherwise unsuitable veins.

When considering the anatomy of the deltopectoral groove, studies from PORTAS 1–3 have shown that the cephalic vein can be visualized with a sufficient diameter in 90% of cases. However, in repeat procedures, recurrences, or cases with anatomical variations, the

Supplementary Information The online version contains supplementary material available at https://doi.org/10.1007/978-3-662-70624-4_13. The videos can be accessed individually by clicking the DOI link in the accompanying figure caption or by scanning this link with the SN More Media App.

R. Hennes (✉)
Klinik für Allgemein-, Viszeral- und Transplantationschirurgie, Universitätsklinikum Heidelberg, Heidelberg, Germany
e-mail: Roland.Hennes@med.uni-heidelberg.de

R. Hennes (ed.), *Port Surgery*, https://doi.org/10.1007/978-3-662-70624-4_13

technical challenge for the surgeon increases. As noted earlier, only small accompanying veins of the pectoralis muscle or other venous branches, typically measuring between 0.5 mm and 1 mm in diameter, are often available. As these delicate veins have to be handled with care, standard surgical instruments no longer suffice. Amicrosurgical approach is required, including surgical loupes with 2- to 3-fold magnification.

In order to apply a microsurgical technique via venous cutdown for port placement, it is necessary to address the modified Seldinger technique first, as it is the prerequisite for employing a microsurgical approach.

The modified Seldinger technique ideally complements the standardized approach via venous cutdown.

In Fig. 13.1, the surgical site is shown with a vein approximately 0.5 mm in diameter, in direct comparison to the port catheter. The marked discrepancy between the vein and the port catheter is clearly visible. For such small veins, we select a guidewire with a tip measuring 0.3 mm.

After looping the vein, it is opened microsurgically using venous cutdown technique aided by surgical loupes (Fig. 13.2). Care must be taken to avoid excessive traction on the vein and accidental tearing.

A 0.3 mm guidewire is then introduced and advanced under fluoroscopic guidance to the right atrium (Fig. 13.3).

This is usually accomplished without difficulty. If branches are encountered, various maneuvers can be used to guide the wire to the right atrium.

▶ **Practical Tip** By extending the arm on the operative side, the vein can often be straightened, making it easier to advance the guidewire. Simple maneuvers such as turning the head are also often helpful in maneuvering the guidewire.

After advancing the guidewire and confirming correct positioning in front of the atrium (Fig. 13.4), a sheath is then introduced over the guidewire (Fig. 13.5). The sheath is advanced under fluoroscopic guidance through the subclavian vein toward the atrium using a rotating motion. It has proven effective not to push the sheath beyond the medial third of the clavicle to avoid injury to the superior vena cava. Before advancing the sheath with the dilator, the distal ligature should be tied to prevent peripheral bleeding. Such small veins, with diameters up to 1 mm, may tear or rupture after insertion of the dilator and sheath. Our extensive practical experience has demonstrate no significant bleeding however.

After placement of the sheath and dilator, the guidewire and dilator are withdrawn and the port catheter is inserted (Fig. 13.6).

Under fluoroscopic guidance, the port catheter is then advanced further to the atrium of the heart (Fig. 13.7).

The sheath is then removed and the catheter is trimmed to the desired length. The following steps are performed as described in Chap. 10 (venae sectio of the cephalic vein), until completion of the procedure.

The surgical procedure of the modified Seldinger technique can be viewed as a video (Fig. 13.8).

This approach has proven safe for port catheter implantation, particularly in small veins or challenging anatomical conditions. The technique accommodates various modifications—for instance, advancing the port catheter solely over the guidewire, where a tapered catheter tip has demonstrated particular effectiveness. However, few manufacturers offer tapered tips, which are technically feasible only with polyurethane catheters. This represents a disadvantage of silicone catheters, which allow at most a rounded tip. The tapered port catheter tip facilitates easy insertion—particularly in small veins—and, with the modified Seldinger technique, enables introduction without a dilator or sheath.

Even with a sufficiently large-lumen cephalic vein, it is not uncommon for the inserted port catheter to deviate into a branch that does not lead to the atrium of the heart. In such cases, the guidewire can facilitate navigation. All of the mentioned techniques require intraoperative

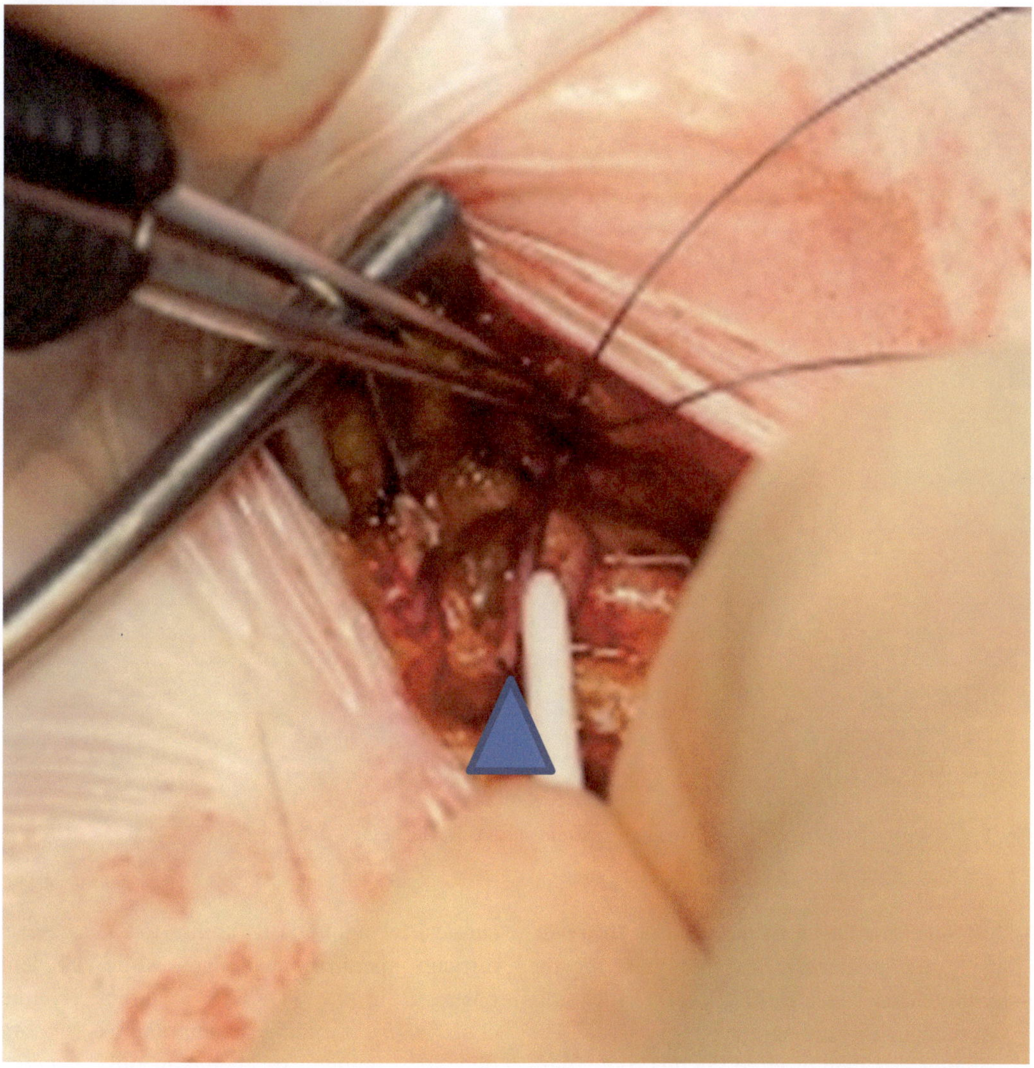

Fig. 13.1 Disproportion between vein diameter 0.5 mm and catheter (6.6 Fr). The tip of the blue triangle points to the vein. (© R. Hennes; all rights reserved)

use of fluoroscopy. ECG-guided techniques for confirming port catheter position preclude such methods and substantially limit surgical options. In our experience, however, ECG guidance remains advisable for port placement during pregnancy. The much-discussed intraoperative radiation exposure is very low with modern fluoroscopy units; especially in oncology patients, who routinely undergo CT scans and other imaging, the radiation exposure from fluoroscopic position control is negligible by comparison. Radiation exposure for staff is also very low and does not represent a relevant risk, as dosimeter evaluations of OR personnel during port procedures over several years have shown.

Case Example: Thrombosis of the Subclavian Vein

Occasionally, special situations arise, as shown in Figs. 13.9, 13.10, and 13.11, where thrombosis precluded implantation via the

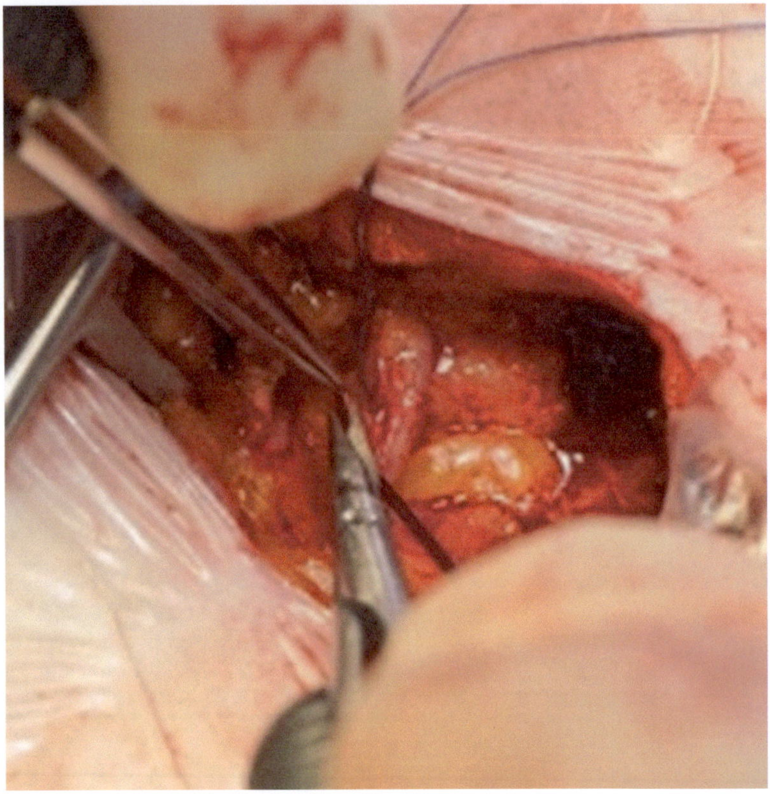

Fig. 13.2 Venous cutdown using microsurgical instruments. (© R. Hennes; all rights reserved)

left subclavian vein to the atrium. However, using the guidewire, a viable path for the port catheter was identified via the right side, as seen in the radiograph (Fig. 13.10). The catheter was then inserted via this route, with excellent function. ◀

However, these techniques require greater surgical experience and should be performed by an experienced surgeon. To successfully perform these techniques in all situations, guidewires of varying stiffness are required. Additionally, a torque device mounted on the guidewire has proven useful for safe navigation.

The use of the modified Seldinger technique in combination with a microsurgical approach is certainly more complex than standard port implantation. The advantage of this surgical technique is its ability to manage even difficult operative challenges while, as demonstrated in the PORTAS-3 studies (Hüttner et al. 2015), avoiding pneumothorax—a complication unique to percutaneous puncture methods in port implantation. In our view, the modified Seldinger technique warrants routine use, including as a microsurgical procedure when needed. The modestly longer operative time is a worthwhile trade-off to minimize patient risks and complications.

These techniques can be applied to all central venous catheters. These techniques are also applied to Hickman catheter placement. Particularly with large-bore or double-lumen Hickman catheters, the modified Seldinger technique—featuring open guidewire insertion followed by dilator and sheath use—proves highly

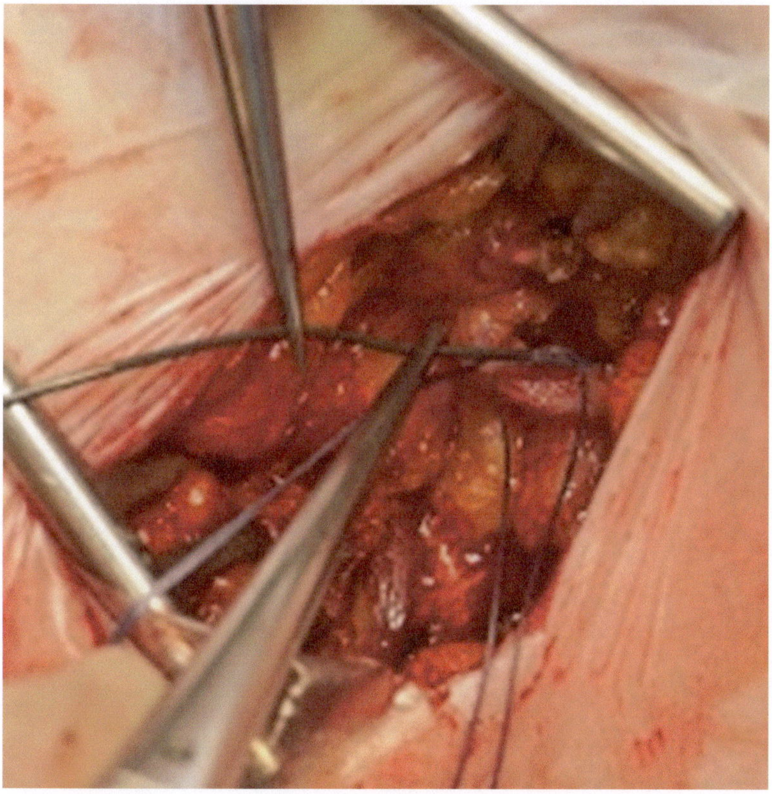

Fig. 13.3 Insertion of the guidewire into the vein. (© R. Hennes; all rights reserved)

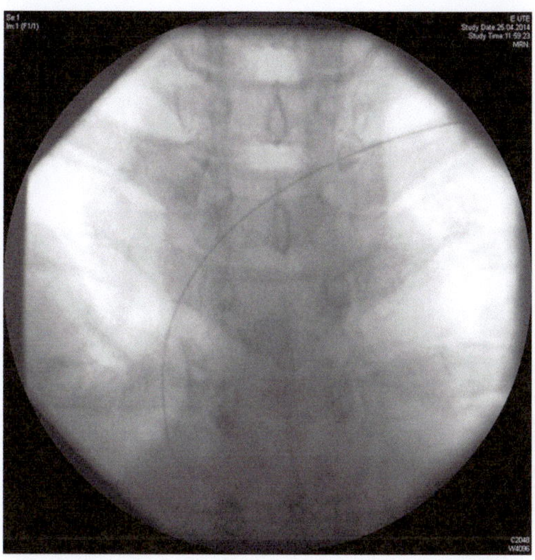

Fig. 13.4 After insertion of the guidewire, radiographic control and fluoroscopic documentation. (© R. Hennes; all rights reserved)

effective. As with port implantation, no percutaneous puncture is required, enabling straightforward, complication-free feeding catheter placement..

Figure 13.12 shows the materials we use for the microsurgical technique: guidewires, sheath, microsurgical instruments, and surgical loupes.

We recommend learning and establishing this technique as a standard adjunct procedure, as it reduces intraoperative complications, streamlines the surgical process, and prevents unnecessary termination of operations.

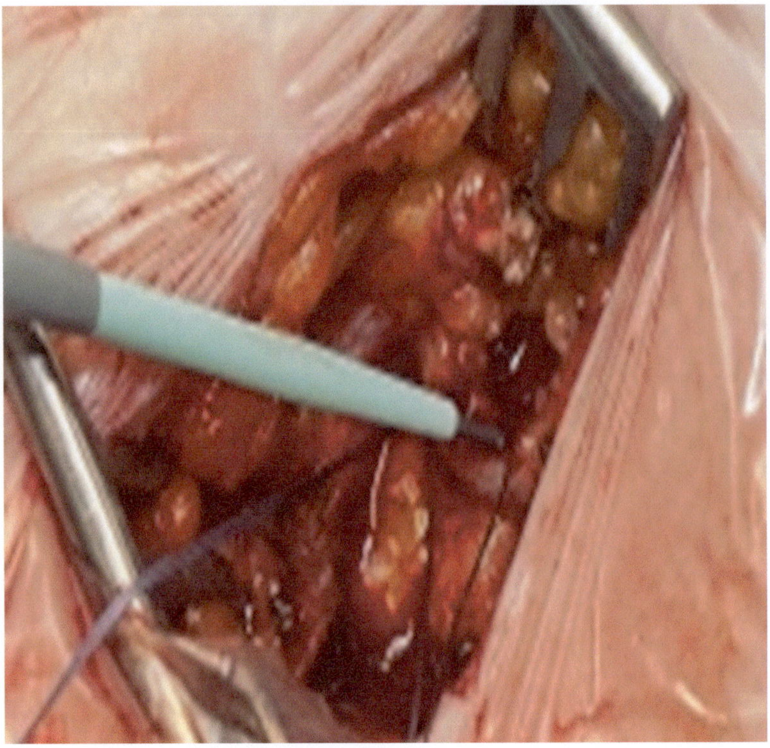

Fig. 13.5 Insertion of the sheath with dilator over the guidewire. (© R. Hennes; all rights reserved)

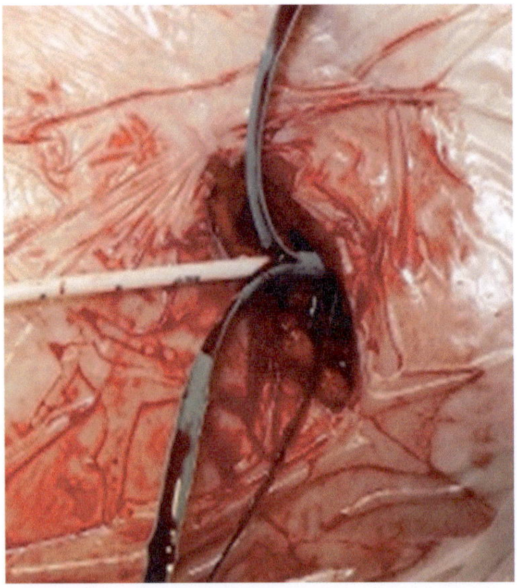

Fig. 13.6 Insertion of the port catheter through the sheath after removal of the dilator and guidewire. The sheath is then removed. (© R. Hennes; all rights reserved)

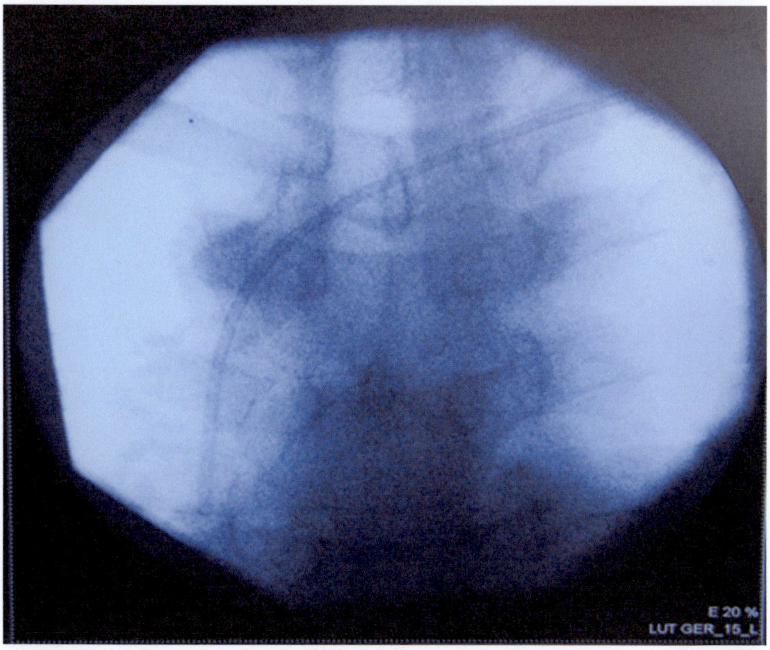

Fig. 13.7 Advancement of the port catheter to approximately one vertebral body below the tracheal bifurcation. (© R. Hennes; all rights reserved)

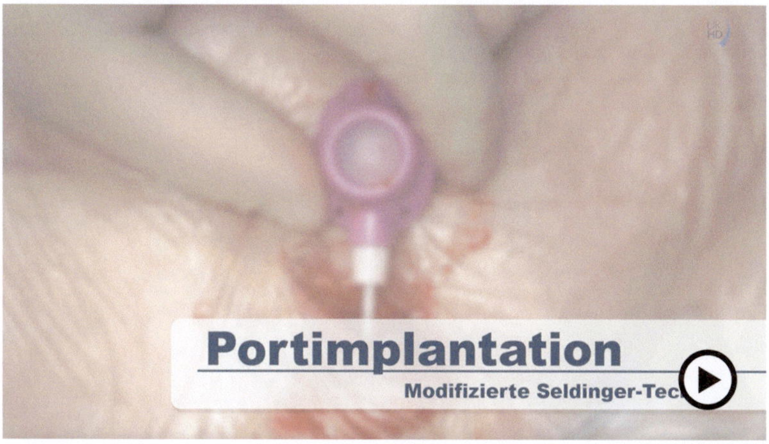

Fig. 13.8 Port implantation using the modified Seldinger technique. (© R. Hennes; all rights reserved). Please use the SN More Media app to play this video and scan the following URL: ▸ https://doi.org/10.1007/000-hgm

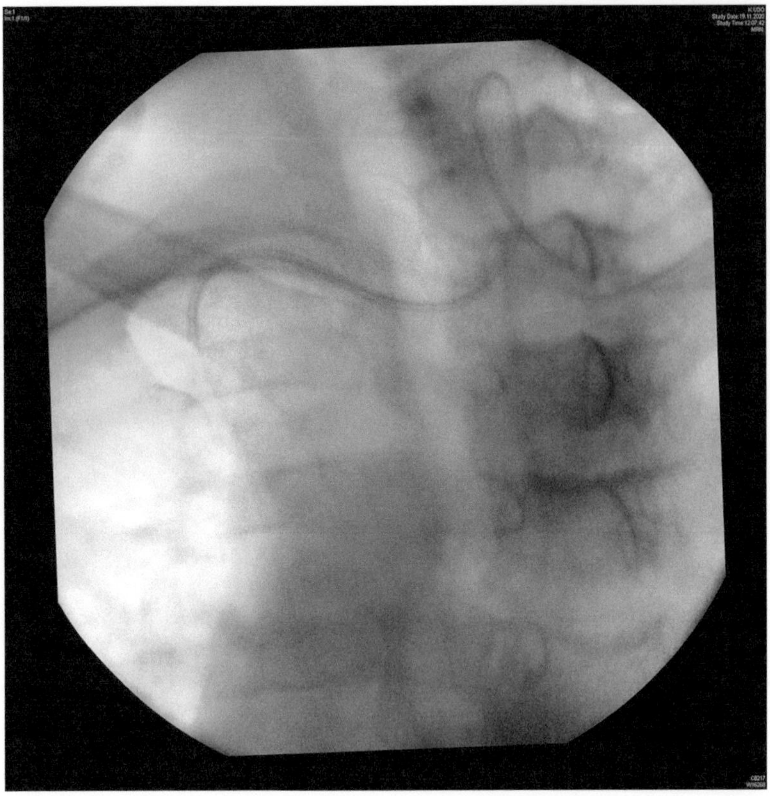

Fig. 13.9 Case example: Overcoming a thrombosis in the area of the left subclavian vein with "loop formation" via collaterals and redirecting to the right subclavian vein. (© R. Hennes; all rights reserved)

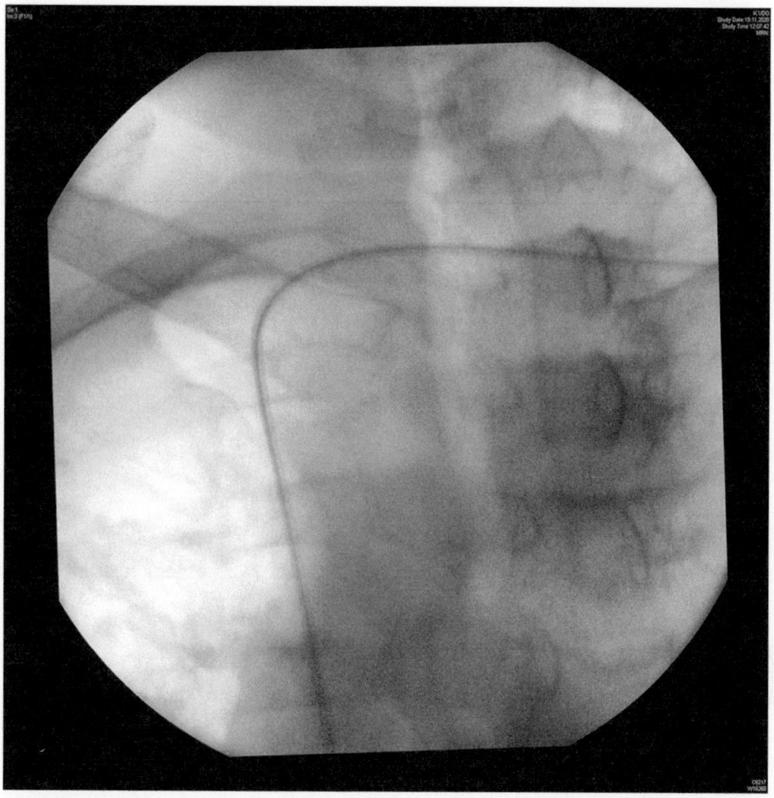

Fig. 13.10 Correction of the loop formation and straightening of the guidewire via the left cephalic and subclavian veins to the right side. The port catheter was then easily inserted over the guidewire. (© R. Hennes; all rights reserved)

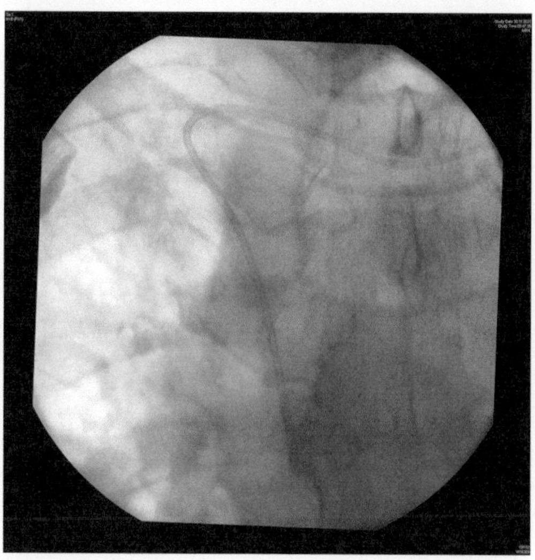

Fig. 13.11 Removal of the guidewire and final placement of the port catheter. (© R. Hennes; all rights reserved)

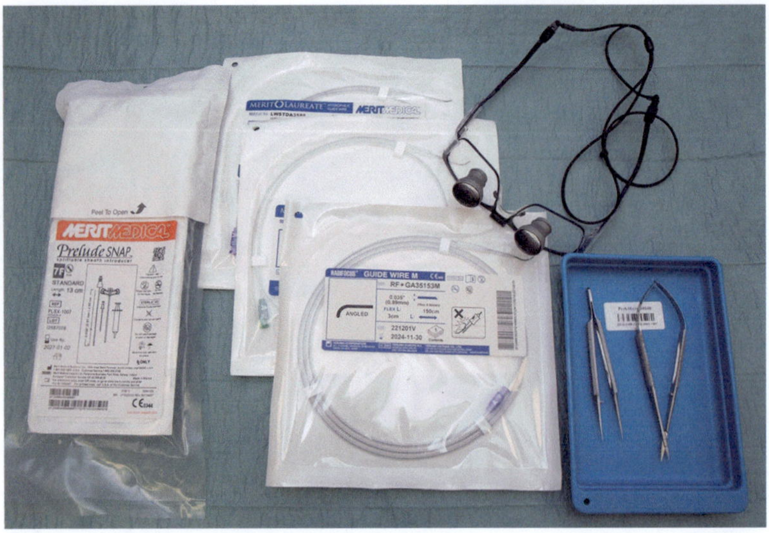

Fig. 13.12 Materials for the microsurgical technique: sheath, guidewires, microsurgical instruments, and surgical loupes. (© R. Hennes; all rights reserved)

References

Knebel P, Fischer L, Huesing J et al (2009) Randomized clinical trial of a modified Seldinger technique for open central venous cannulation for implantable access devices. Br J Surg 96:159–165

Knebel P, Lopez-Benitez R, Fischer L et al (2011) Insertion of totally implantable venous access devices: an expertise-based, randomized, controlled trial (NCT00600444). Ann Surg 253:1111–1117

Hüttner FJ, Bruckner T, Alldinger I et al (2015) Frequency of pneumothorax and haemothorax after primary open versus closed implantation strategies for insertion of a totally implantable venous access port in oncological patients: study protocol for a randomised controlled trial. Trials 16:128

Polychronidis G, Hennes R, Engerer C et al (2017) Use of a hydrophilic coating wire reduces significantly the rate of central vein punctures and the incidence of pneumothorax in totally implantable access port (TIAP) surgery. BMC Surg 17:131

Interventional Transhepatic and Translumbar Port Placement

14

De-Hua Chang

▶ Central venous catheters have become indispensable in medicine for the care of patients requiring long-term venous access. They provide a safe and repeatedly accessible vascular route, often sparing patients the discomfort of difficult peripheral vein punctures. However, the increasing use of central venous catheters has been accompanied by a rising incidence of catheter-related thrombosis. Long-term catheters are responsible for 10% of all deep vein thromboses in adults, and in children, the proportion is as high as 50–80% (Citla Sridhar D et al. 2020). Multiple peripheral or central chronic vascular occlusions often present a significant challenge for re-implantation of a port catheter via the upper extremity. Various minimally invasive techniques and alternative access routes have been developed for cases where conventional implantation is no longer feasible. The most frequently described alternatives in the literature include the common femoral vein, hepatic vein, and inferior vena cava. (Denny DF 2011; Grözinger G et al. 2018). Due to lower patient comfort and a high infection rate, the common femoral vein should be reserved for temporary access, and avoided for long-term therapy whenever possible (Ge X et al. 2012). The following provides a detailed description of transhepatic and translumbar port implantation.

D.-H. Chang (✉)
Radiologie und Nuklearmedizin, Kantonsspital Luzern, Luzern, Switzerland
e-mail: de-hua.chang@luks.ch

14.1 Transhepatic Port Placement

Prior to the intervention, the target vein for puncture is identified using ultrasound. Typically, the right hepatic vein is best suited for port placement due to its long, straight course. The procedure can be performed under analgosedation. Extensive local anesthesia is administered along the access route up to the liver capsule. A skin incision is then made. A Chiba needle (21–22 gauge, 15 cm long) is inserted under ultrasound guidance subcostally or in the area of the caudal third of the liver (10th–12th intercostal space) along the mid-right axillary line. The puncture direction runs parallel to the ribs to access the right hepatic vein at the shallowest possible angle. Correct needle position is confirmed via contrast injection, followed by guidewire advancement into the right atrium. (Fig. 14.1). The guidewire is then exchanged for a stiff exchange wire via a 4-F sheath or dilator. After predilation of the tract, a peel-away sheath is introduced. The port catheter is advanced through the sheath. The tip of the catheter should initially be placed in the right atrium and

R. Hennes (ed.), *Port Surgery*, https://doi.org/10.1007/978-3-662-70624-4_14

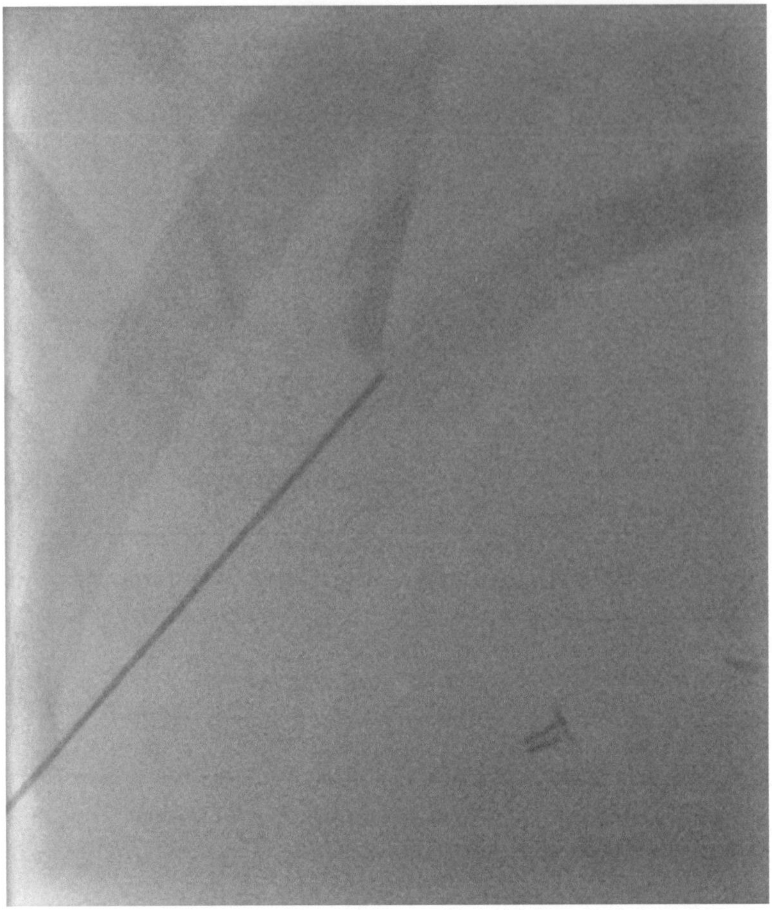

Fig. 14.1 A contrast injection through the needle confirms correct positioning in the right hepatic vein

only withdrawn into the inferior vena cava after removal of the sheath. (Advancing the catheter after sheath removal is significantly more difficult due to frictional resistance.)

The skin incision for preparing the port pocket is made under local anesthesia in the ventrolateral upper abdomen, below the costal margin. Two absorbable anchoring sutures are placed on the fascia of the external oblique muscle. The port catheter is then tunneled subcutaneously into the port pocket. The catheter is connected to the port chamber, and patency is checked by aspiration. The system is flushed with saline and may additionally be locked with heparin (500 IU). At the end of the procedure, the port chamber is secured to the fascia using the prepared anchoring sutures, and the wound is closed. The position of the catheter and port chamber is shown in Figs. 14.2 and 14.3.

Dislocation of the catheter in the form of looping between the abdominal wall and liver capsule can occur, especially in the early period, due to respiratory excursions. Therefore, verification of correct intravascular position before each infusion (aspiration of blood, ultrasound, or X-ray/fluoroscopy) is absolutely essential.

14.2 Translumbar Port Placement

The procedure is performed with the patient in the prone position under general anesthesia. CT-guided puncture with a 21–22 gauge needle is initiated above the right iliac crest and passes

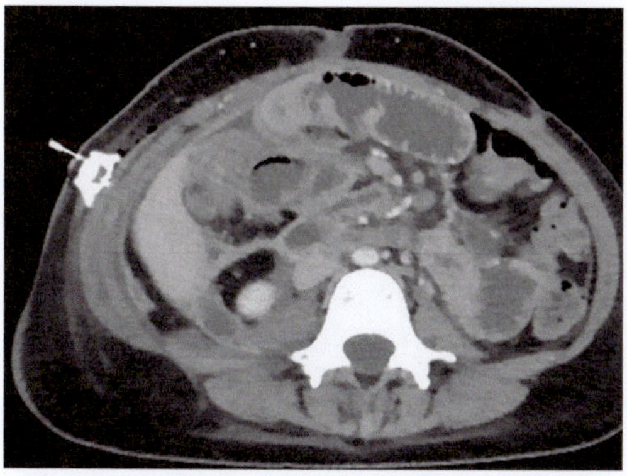

Fig. 14.2 Axial contrast-enhanced computed tomography: The port chamber is fixed to the fascia of the external oblique muscle

through the upper portion of the psoas muscle. The inferior vena cava is penetrated below the entry of the renal veins. Care should be taken to direct the needle slightly cranially to avoid kinking of the catheter at the entry into the inferior vena cava (Fig. 14.4). After establishing access to the inferior vena cava, the guidewire is inserted, and the patient is transferred to the angiography suite.

In-house, puncture of the inferior vena cava is performed using cone-beam CT in the angiography suite. This allows the procedure to be carried carried out in one room only without the need to reposition the patient.

Guided by fluoroscopy, the needle is removed. The guidewire is then exchanged for a stiff exchange wire via a 4-F sheath or dilator. The subsequent steps are performed analogous to the transhepatic port placement (Section 14.1). The port chamber is implanted at the ventrolateral upper abdomen below the costal margin, allowing the catheter to run subcutaneously dorsally along the right flank.

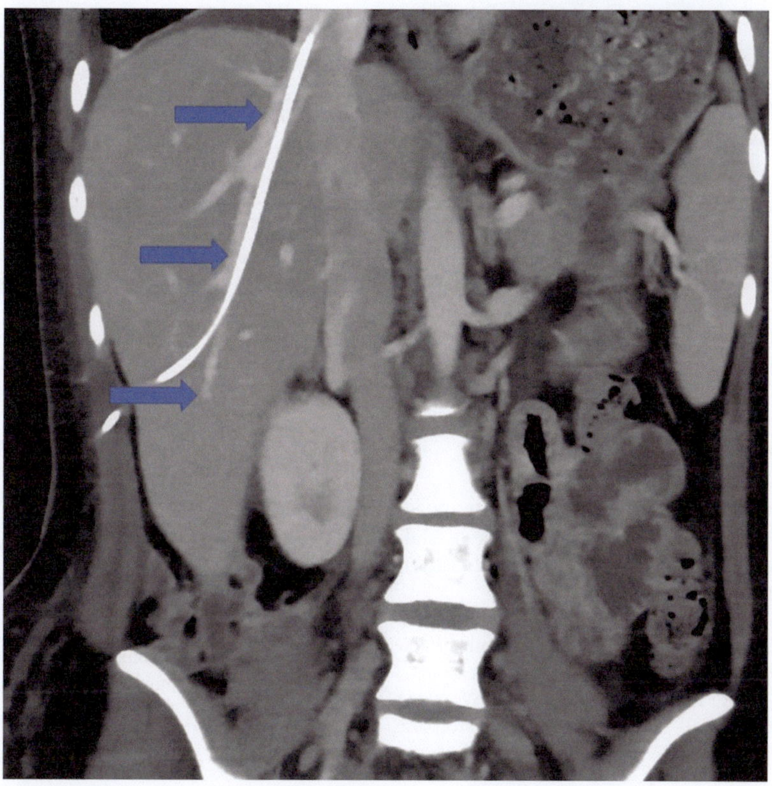

Fig. 14.3 Contrast-enhanced computed tomography (coronal reconstruction): port catheter inserted via the right hepatic vein (arrows)

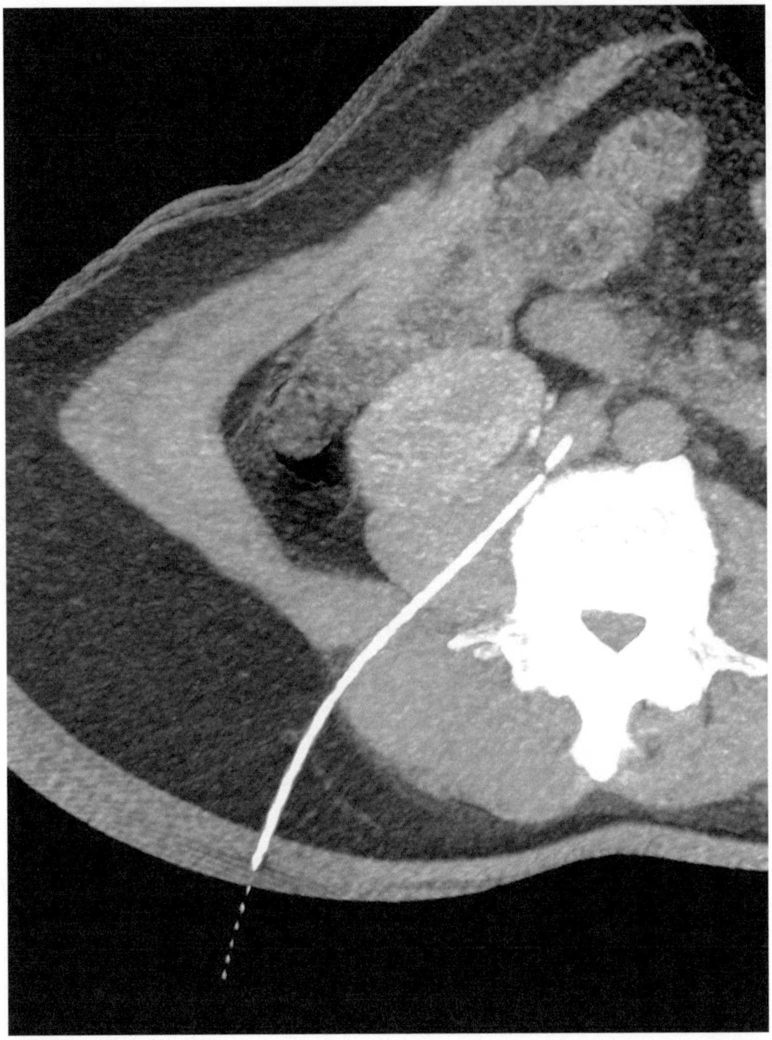

Fig. 14.4 Contrast-enhanced computed tomography (oblique reconstruction): port catheter inserted translumbar via the inferior vena cava

References

Citla Sridhar D, Abou-Ismail MY, Ahuja SP (2020) Central venous catheter-related thrombosis in children and adults. Thromb Res 187:103–112. https://doi.org/10.1016/j.thromres.2020.01.017

Denny DF Jr (2011) Venous access salvage techniques. Tech Vasc Interv Radiol 14(4):225–32. https://doi.org/10.1053/j.tvir.2011.05.006

Ge X, Cavallazzi R, Li C, Pan SM, Wang YW, Wang FL (2012): Central venous access sites for the prevention of venous thrombosis, stenosis and infection. Cochrane Database Syst Rev. 14(3):CD004084. https://doi.org/10.1002/14651858.CD004084.pub3

Grözinger G, Grosse U, Syha R, Hoffmann R, Partovi S, Nikolaou K, Stahl S, Königsrainer A, Thiel K, Thiel C (2018) CT-guided translumbar placement of permanent catheters in the inferior vena cava: description of the technique with technical success and complications data. Cardiovasc Intervent Radiol 41(9):1356–1362. https://doi.org/10.1007/s00270-018-1961-9

Performance of Port Explantation and Management of Complications

15

Roland Hennes

> ▶ Port explantation is often underestimated as a "minor" and insignificant procedure. Ports left in situ for more than five years can lead to extensive vascular adhesions. This can pose significant surgical challenges, demanding a nuanced approach and meticulous technique.

Port explantation is is the procedure required for removal of a port catheter and may be indicated for, a wide range of indications. A study conducted by the Study Center of the Department of Surgery at Heidelberg University Hospital examined the indications for port explantation in 438 patients, of whom 385 were included in the study (Fischer et al. 2008). Infectious complications were the primary reason (46.2%) for explantation. This was followed by completion of oncologic therapy in 129 cases (33.5%), 44 cases of thrombosis (11.4%), and port dysfunction in 22 cases (5.7%). In 12 patients (3.1%) reason for explantation was not specified.

(Figs. 15.1 and 15.2). In such cases surgical revision and port explantation is warrented (Walser 2012).

In long-term indwelling port catheters remaining in situ for over five years, material fatigue may develop, such as corrosion at the catheter-port chamber junction (Fig. 15.3). More peripherally located extravasations may arise from tears in the catheter material, as seen in arm ports (Figs. 15.4 and 15.5). Another indication is a pronounced sheath thrombus (Fig. 15.6) that completely encases the catheter, rendering blood aspiration and flow impossible. Removal may also be requested by the patient, in which case thorough counseling on the port's benefits and functions is essential, including the often-overlooked utility of high-pressure ports for CT and MRI contrast administration.

Overall, the indication for port explantation should be carefully made. We strongly discourage early port explantation immediately after completing the first course of chemotherapy, as the disease trajectory and recovery remain uncertain, potentially necessitating future use. Thorough patient counseling is essential to prevent premature removal, which could require reimplantation—and thus another surgical procedure—during subsequent chemotherapy.

Supplementary Information The online version contains supplementary material available at https://doi.org/10.1007/978-3-662-70624-4_15. The videos can be accessed individually by clicking the DOI link in the accompanying figure caption or by scanning this link with the SN More Media App.

R. Hennes (✉)
Klinik für Allgemein-, Viszeral- und Transplantationschirurgie, Universitätsklinikum Heidelberg, Heidelberg, Germany
e-mail: Roland.Hennes@med.uni-heidelberg.de

R. Hennes (ed.), *Port Surgery*, https://doi.org/10.1007/978-3-662-70624-4_15

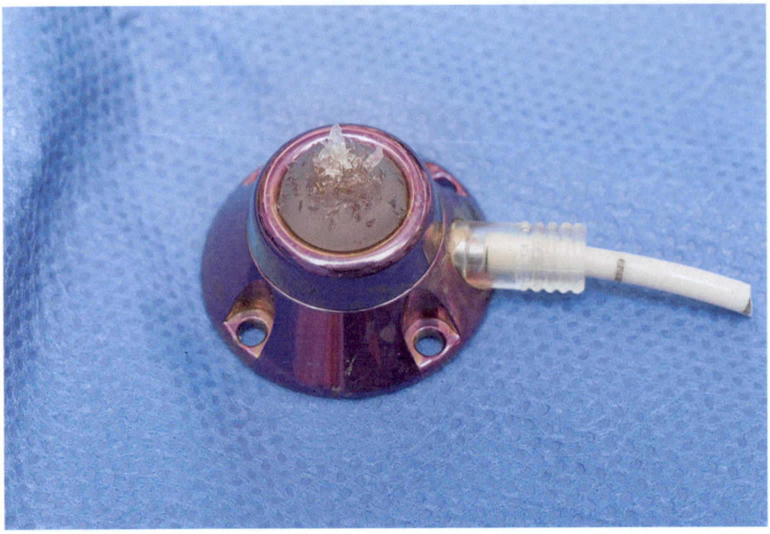

Fig. 15.1 Destruction of the silicone membrane due to incorrect puncture technique and inappropriate needle selection. (© R. Hennes; all rights reserved)

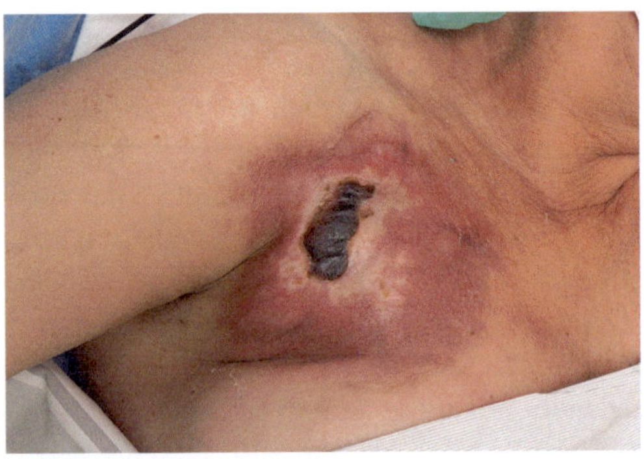

Fig. 15.2 Extravasation following chemotherapy administration with skin necrosis. (© R. Hennes; all rights reserved)

Another indication for explantation is when the port catheter has remained in situ for more than five years (see Chap. 3—Materials for port procedures). At this stage, material fatigue may manifest, increasing the risk of catheter fracture and related complications; in such cases, replacement via a modified Seldinger technique is recommended and typically straightforward. The surgical procedure can be viewed in the video *Portexplanation* (Fig. 15.7).

15.1 Surgical Procedure for Standardized Port Explantation

1. After locating the port chamber—typically straightforward via the prior surgical scar—a spindle-shaped excision of the scar is performed in the operative field, such as in the deltopectoral groove. Port explantation offers an opportunity to improve cosmesis through scar revision. This step is performed routinely(Figs. 15.8 and 15.9).
2. After removal of the scar, the port catheter is routinely exposed and should be removed first. Since the catheter is often "hidden" within the scar tissue, the easiest way to locate it is to identify the catheter connection to the port chamber and lift it with a clamp (Fig. 15.10). The port catheter can then be exposed over a short distance using a monopolar electrosurgical knife.
3. Once the port catheter is exposed, it can be removed by simply pulling it out, if necessary with a clamp (Fig. 15.11). The port catheter is removed first because sharp dissection

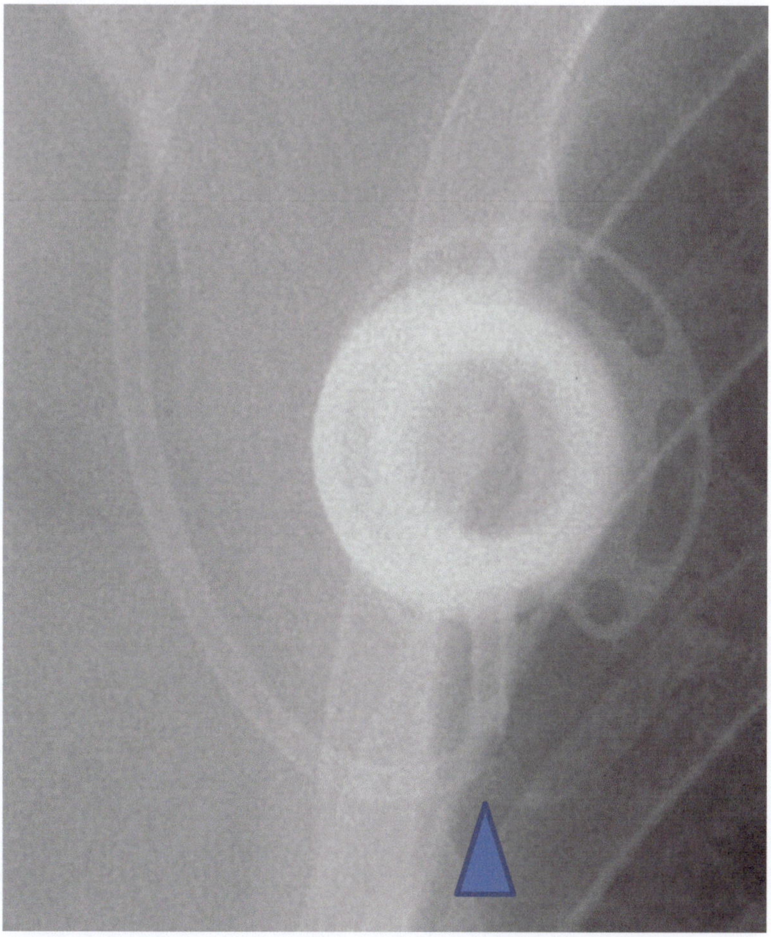

Fig. 15.3 Fracture at the catheter junction due to material fatigue. (© R. Hennes; all rights reserved)

through scar tissue risks transecting it, potentially allowing migration into the venous system and necessitating complex interventional retrieval, such as from the pulmonary circulation.

> **Practical Tip** Removal of the port catheter from the vein should be performed as the first step during port explantation, before removing the port chamber. Otherwise, there is a risk of severing and central migration of the catheter!

4. After the port catheter has been removed from the tissue, adhesions around the port chamber are released using an electrosurgical knife or scalpel. Care must be taken to identify any sutures, which may be either absorbable or nonabsorbable depending on the implantation technique. Nonabsorbable sutures must be located, divided, and removed from the surrounding tissue (Fig. 15.12). Once all adhesions have been released, the entire port system can be removed.

> **Practical Tip** If the catheter cannot be easily removed from the vein, first check whether it is fixed to the cephalic vein or surrounding tissue with a non-absorbable subcutaneous suture. This requires exposing the catheter along its visible extracorporeal course.

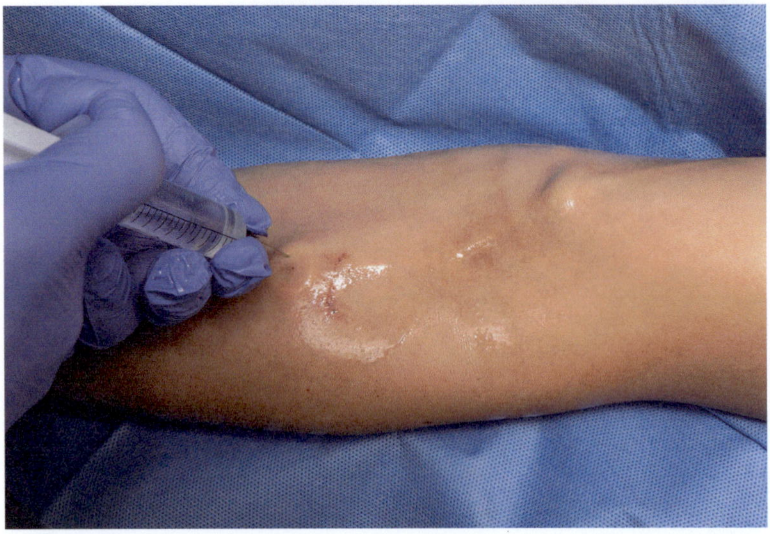

Fig. 15.4 Visualization of extravasation due to catheter fracture in the antecubital fossa of an arm port. (© R. Hennes; all rights reserved)

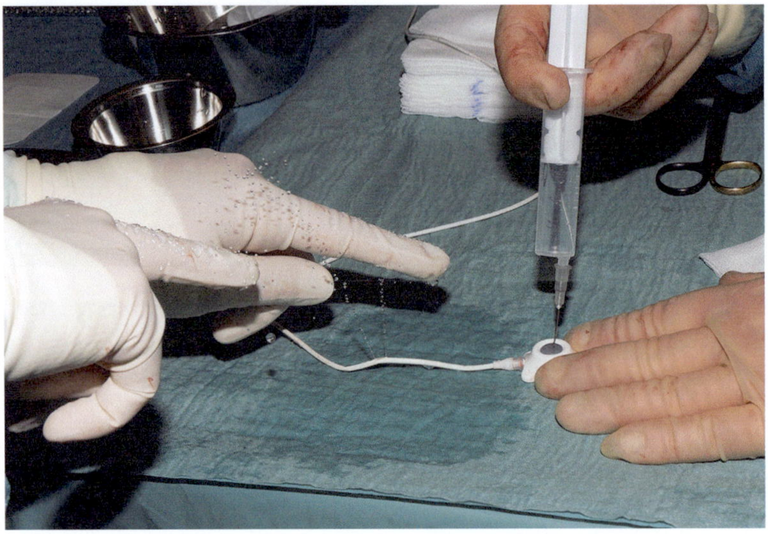

Fig. 15.5 After explantation of the arm port: visualization of the catheter fracture. (© R. Hennes; all rights reserved)

5. The remaining port pocket, with its characteristic epithelialized lining around the port chamber, should not be resected. This avoids unnecessary bleeding and postoperative hematoma formation; the epithelial lining should simply be left in situ.
6. This is followed by thorough irrigation and inspection for hemostasis. Careful control of bleeding is achieved with diathermy. Wound closure can be performed using either a continuous two-layer suture technique or interrupted single stitches, depending on the patient's constitution and the thickness of the subcutaneous fat layer.

The former entry site of the port catheter into the cephalic or subclavian vein does not need to be specifically identified. It is sufficient to place

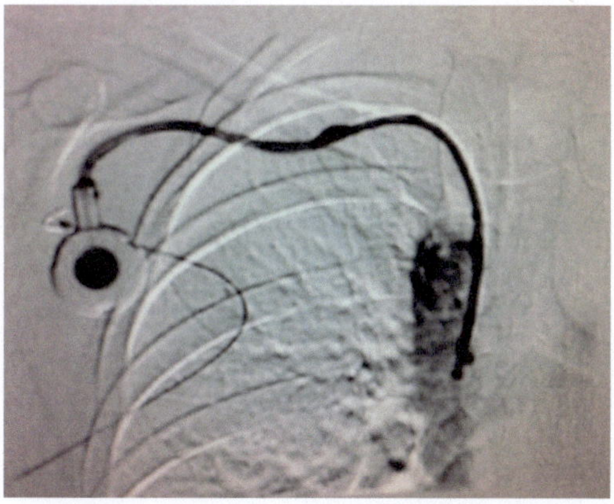

Fig. 15.6 Pronounced sheath thrombus. (© R. Hennes; all rights reserved)

a transfixion suture in this area, which can be done as part of the subcutaneous closure. Due to the "curtain effect" of the tissue, the individual layers shift over one another, preventing secondary bleeding from this area. Meticulous hemostasis and depp subcutaneous sutures obliterating dead space by closing tissue compartments, largely eliminates the risk of postoperative bleeding and hematoma formation.

7. Skin closure is performed with absorbable sutures in cases of unremarkable wound conditions and at the end of therapy. In cases of infection or pus formation around the port chamber, open wound management is indicated (Fig. 15.13).

15.2 Surgical Approach to Adhesions and Complications of Port Explantation

In principle, adhesions of the port catheter system to the surrounding vessel can occur with any port. As a rule, we observe adhesions and encapsulation of the port chamber—more or less pronounced—in all ports after just a few weeks.

These adhesions can be easily released using electrocautery (or a scalpel in the case of titanium ports), allowing the port chamber to be exposed without difficulty (Fig. 15.14).

Intraluminal adhesions of the vessels can present particular challenges.

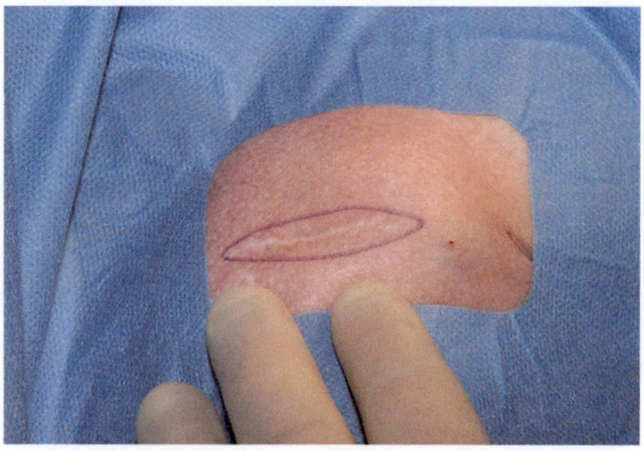

Fig. 15.8 Marking the incision line for spindle-shaped excision of the scar. (© R. Hennes; all rights reserved)

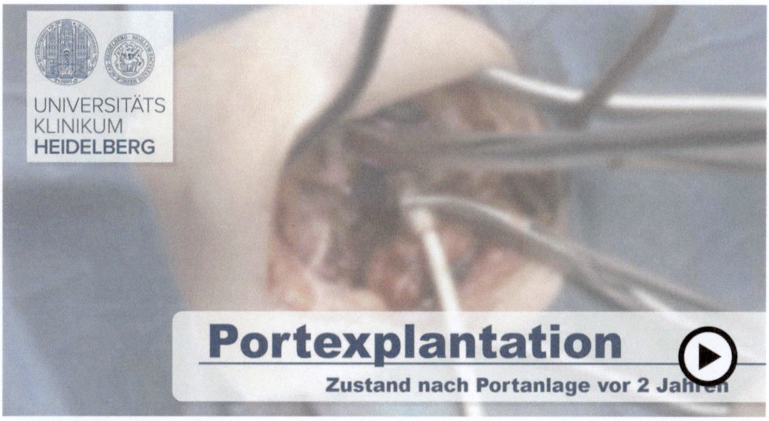

Fig. 15.7 Port explantation. (© R. Hennes; all rights reserved). Please use the SN More Media app to play this video and scan the following URL: ▸ https://doi.org/10.1007/000-hgn.

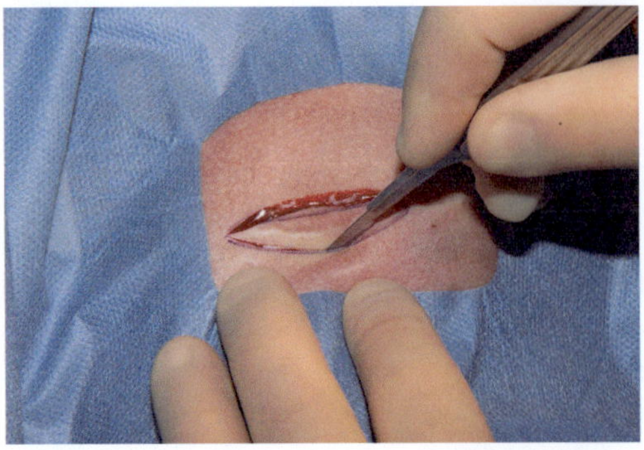

Fig. 15.9 Spindle-shaped excision of the scar. (© R. Hennes; all rights reserved)

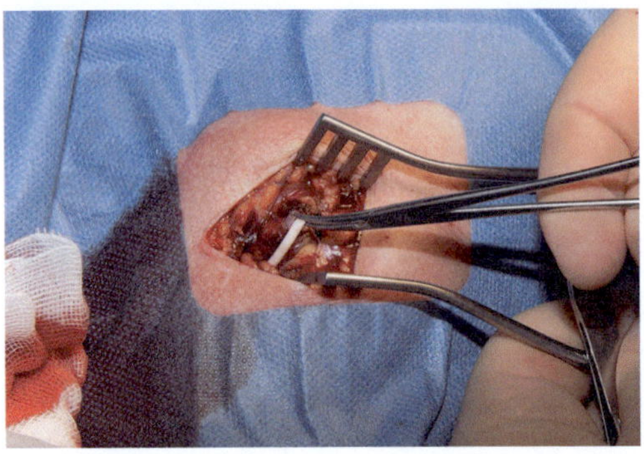

Fig. 15.10 Lifting the catheter at the connection site (© R. Hennes; all rights reserved)

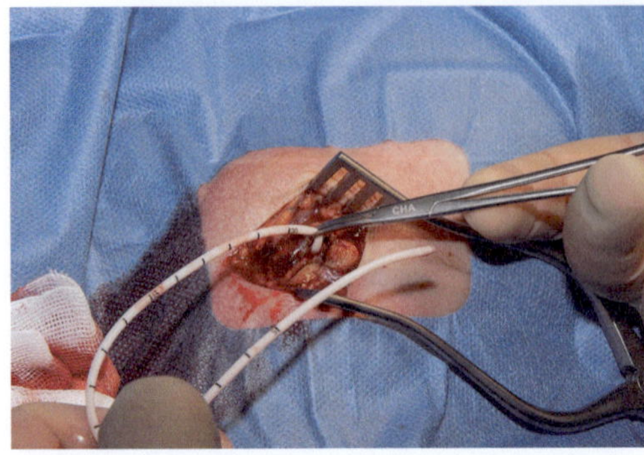

Fig. 15.11 Extraction of the catheter from the vein. (© R. Hennes; all rights reserved)

Significant adhesions to the vessels are most commonly found in ports that have remained in situ for more than five years. As described by Haindl (Chap. 3), material fatigue after five years can cause the port catheter to become brittle, leading not only to adhesion but also to complete tearing during removal.

In this context, it may be helpful to perform a preoperative phlebography to visualize the course of the port catheter, in order to assess the extent of adhesions and plan the explantation procedure. Difficult cases can often be managed successfully through interdisciplinary collaboration, with an interventional radiologist retrieving

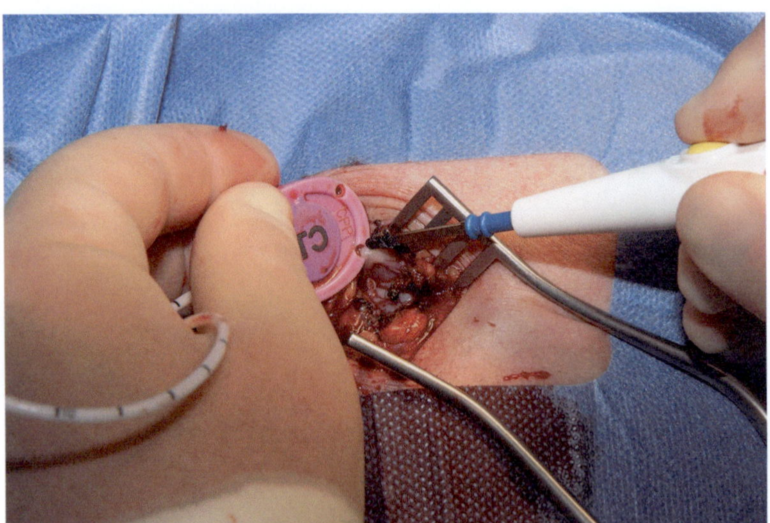

Fig. 15.12 Releasing adhesions around the port chamber with electrocautery. (© R. Hennes; all rights reserved)

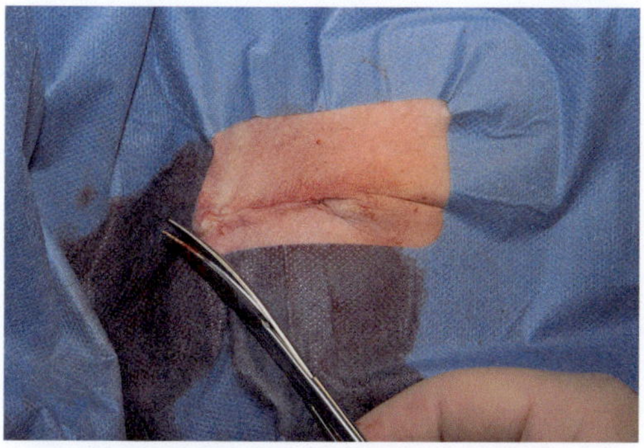

Fig. 15.13 Wound closure with absorbable intracutaneous suture. ()

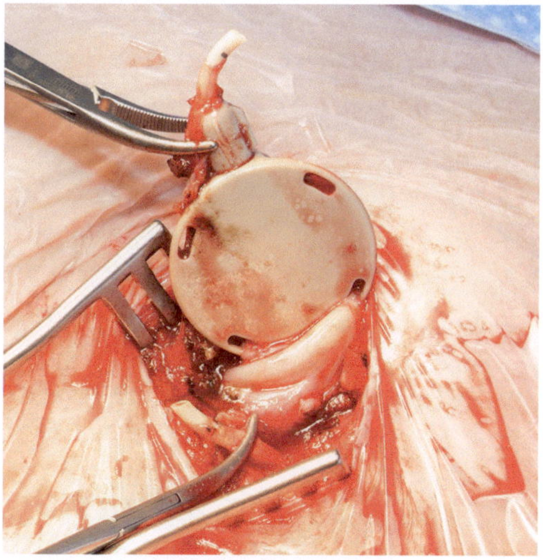

Fig. 15.14 Exposure of the port chamber with its adhesions. ()

the port using a snare.(Figs. 15.15 and 15.16). This technique can also be applied to fractured catheters. For example, this approach was used for an incidentally discovered catheter dislocation into the inferior vena cava two years after port implantation. (Fig. 15.17). Figure 15.18 shows another example of retrieval of a dislocated catheter that had fractured due to material fatigue and was again successfully retrieved interventionally.

If extensive intraluminal adhesions are present along the entire course of the catheter, the decision to attempt definitive catheter removal should be reconsidered.

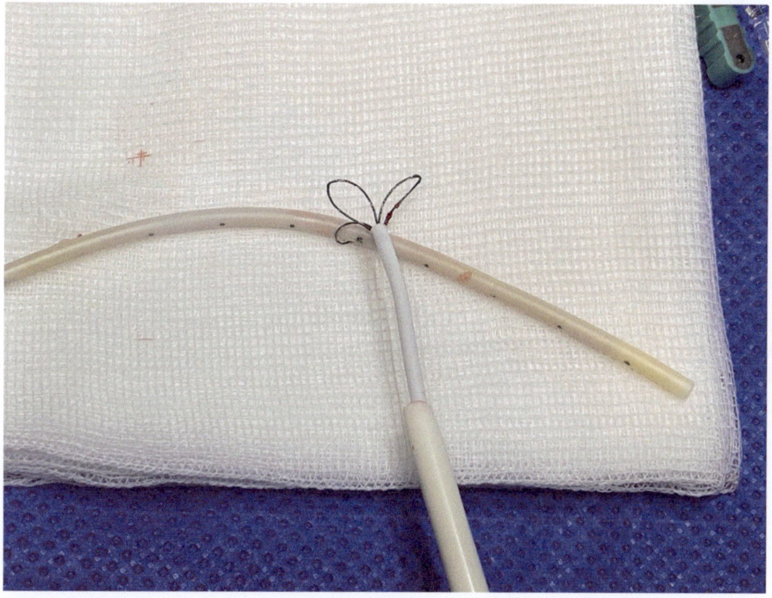

Fig. 15.15 Retrieval of a fractured catheter using a snare. ()

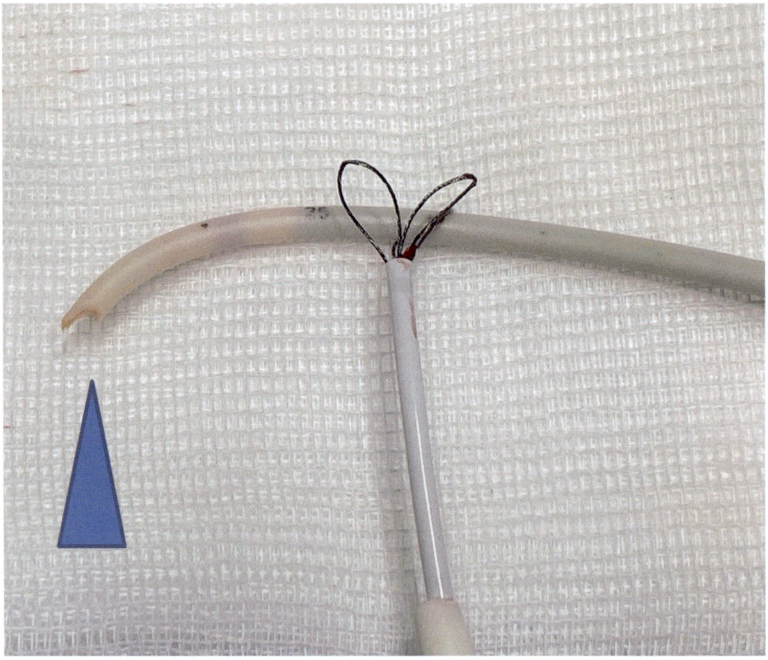

Fig. 15.16 Retrieved port catheter, removed with a snare. The blue triangle indicates the location of the catheter fracture. (© R. Hennes; all rights reserved)

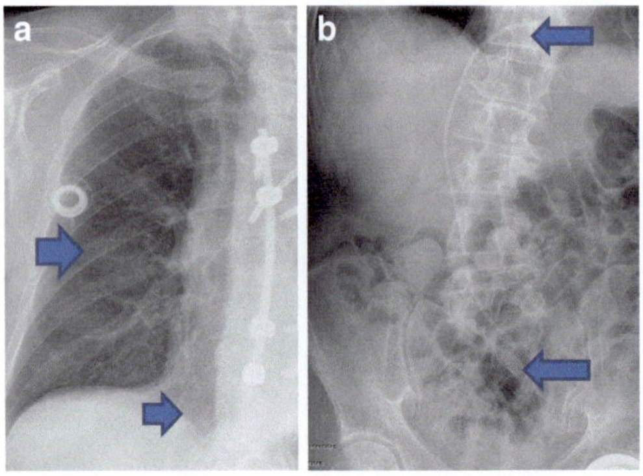

Fig. 15.17 a,b Incidental finding of a catheter dislocated into the inferior vena cava two years after implantation. (© R. Hennes; all rights reserved)

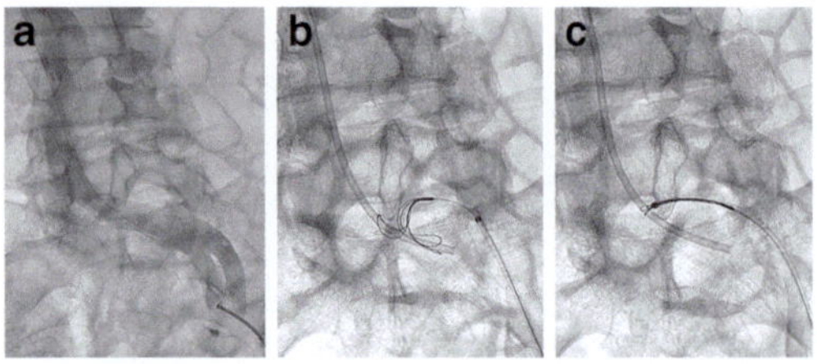

Fig. 15.18 a–c Snaring of the port catheter. Complete removal via an indwelling sheath in the left groin. (© R. Hennes; all rights reserved)

15.3 Port Removal with Insertion of a Guidewire to Stabilize the Port Catheter in Cases of Old Catheter Material

The experience of older catheters becoming brittle and prone to fracture prompted the development of a stabilization technique using an internal guidewire. This allows secure removal with two clamps grasping both the catheter and the intraluminal wire.

Surgical Procedure

Step 1

If the catheter cannot be easily withdrawn intraoperatively and exhibits the typical "rubber band" stretching, it should be stabilized from within using a guidewire. After transection of the port catheter at the level of the chamber and securing it with a clamp, the guidewire is inserted into the catheter under fluoroscopic guidance, thereby stabilizing the catheter from the inside (Figs. 15.14, 15.19 and 15.20).

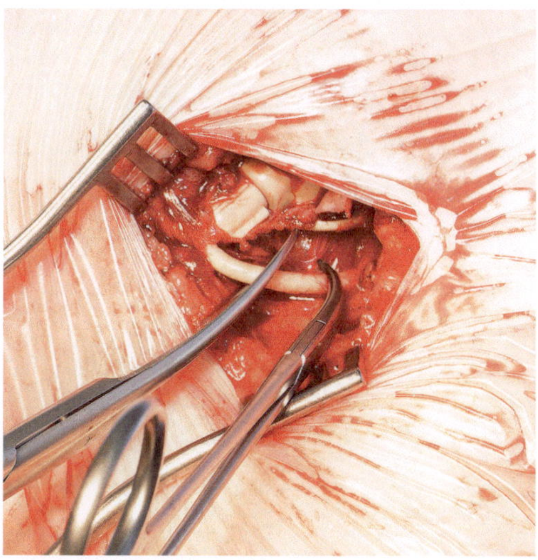

Fig. 15.19 Transection of the catheter at the port chamber. The catheter is first grasped and secured with a clamp. ((© R. Hennes; all rights reserved)

Step 2

Grasp the catheter with two clamps, repositioning them repeatedly at different sites to avoid tearing or breaking the catheter material due to the clamps.

Step 3

The catheter is then slowly extracted using rotational movements, with jerky motions strictly avoided. Gentle, progressive withdrawal—with repeated grip repositioning and rotational loosening—is recommended under fluoroscopic guidance to confirm correct directional movement and release(Fig. 15.21).

Step 4

After catheter removal—often revealing typical fibrin deposits (Fig. 15.22) —careful ligation of the soft tissue at the extraction site is performed. Post-removal bleeding, which may occur due to adherent fibrin, is typically controlled by targeted ligation.

▶ **Practical Tip** For catheters adherent to vessels, intraluminal stabilization with a guidewire can facilitate removal and minimize breakage risk. Such procedures should be performed only by experienced surgeons; if local expertise is insufficient, the catheter should be secured in place and the patient referred to a specialized center.

Case Example: Osseous Adhesion of the Port Catheter to the Clavicle Another rare complication is port catheter adhesion to the clavicle due to periosteal injury following puncture-based insertion (Fig. 15.23) (Hennes and Hofmann 2016). In this case, osseous adhesion necessitated clavicle osteotomy by an orthopedic surgeon to remove surrounding bone and retrieve the fractured port catheter segment, which exhibited extensive adhesions. (Fig. 15.24).

After removal of the catheter, the clavicle was stabilized again with plate osteosynthesis (Fig. 15.25).

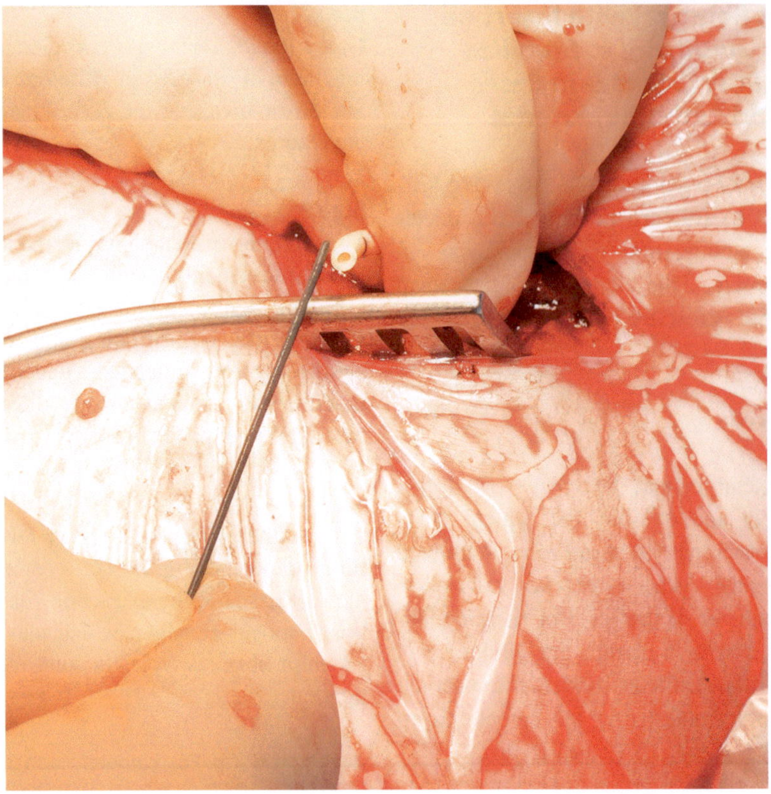

Fig. 15.20 Insertion of a guidewire to stabilize the catheter. (© R. Hennes; all rights reserved)

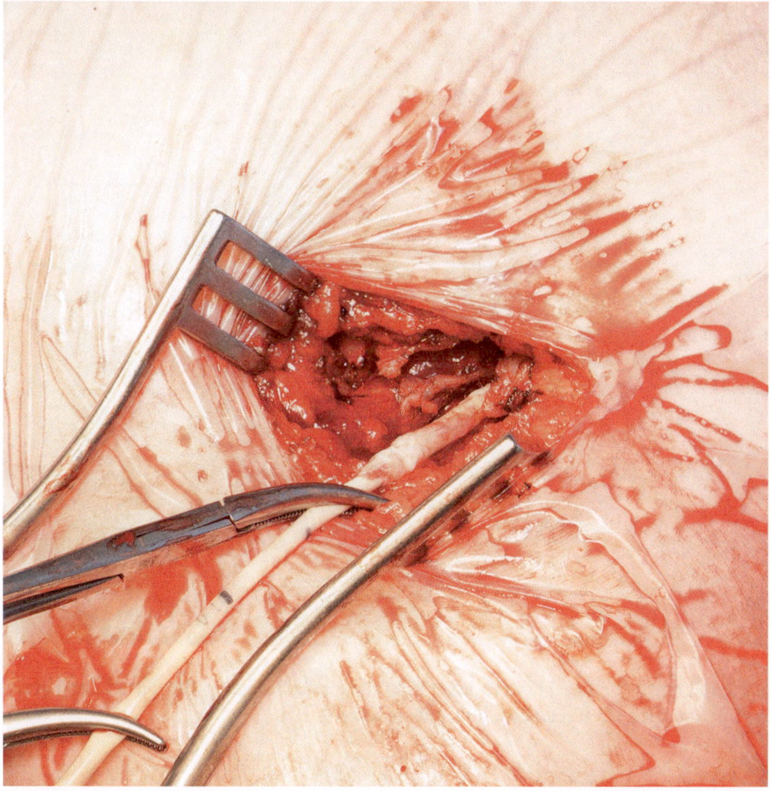

Fig. 15.21 Placement of two clamps on the catheter and the guidewire inside it. The catheter is then withdrawn using rotational movements. (© R. Hennes; all rights reserved)

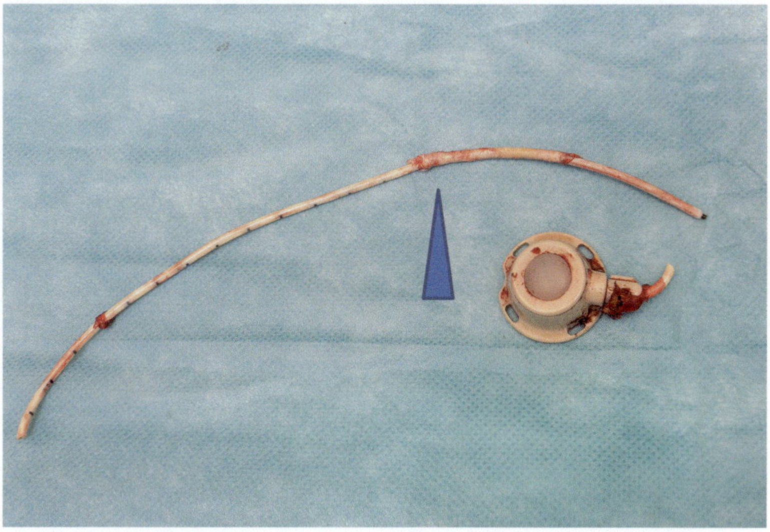

Fig. 15.22 Removed port chamber and port catheter with adherent adhesions. The blue triangle indicates the adhesions around the catheter. (© R. Hennes; all rights reserved)

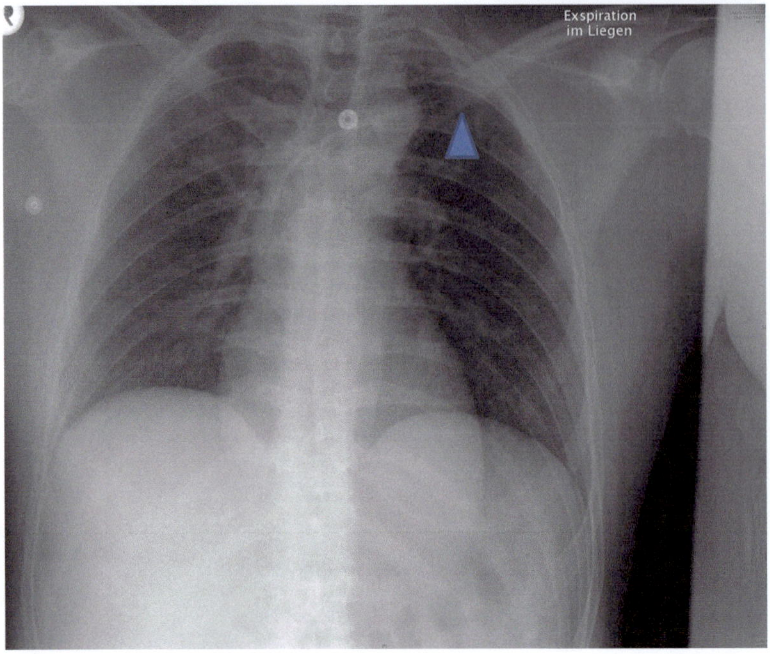

Fig. 15.23 Figure depicting a fractured port catheter with osseous adhesion to the clavicle and periosteum. The blue triangle marks the fracture site. (© R. Hennes; all rights reserved)

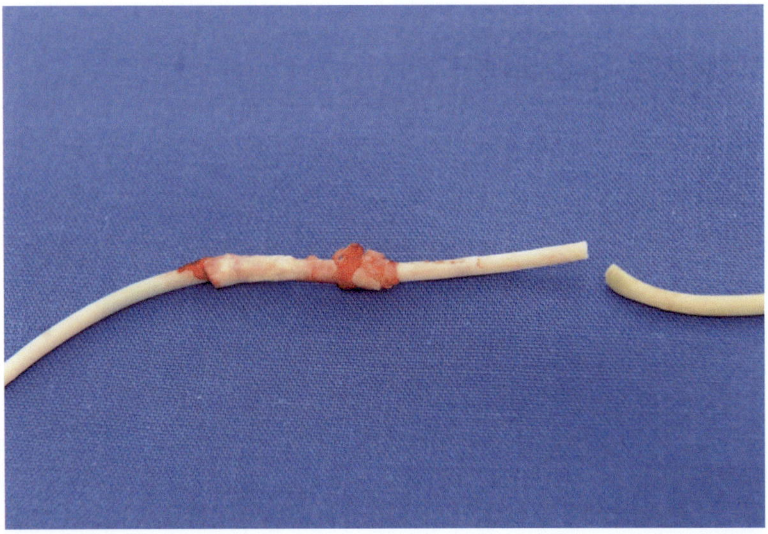

Fig. 15.24 Retrieved catheter after clavicle osteotomy with extensive adhesions. (© R. Hennes; all rights reserved)

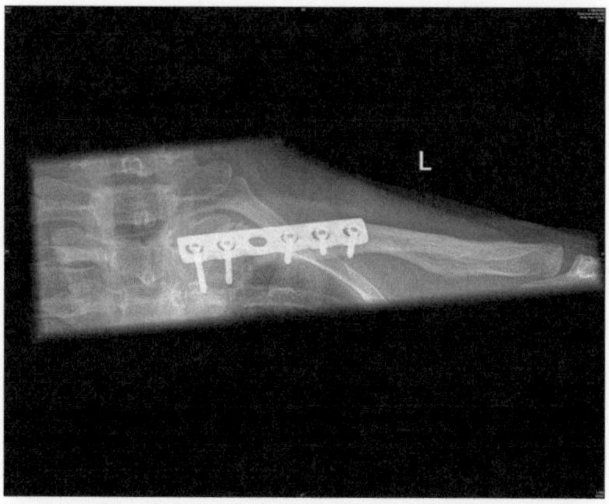

Fig. 15.25 Plate osteosynthesis after clavicle osteotomy and catheter removal. (© R. Hennes; all rights reserved)

References

Fischer L, Knebel P, Schroder S et al (2008) Reasons for explantation of totally implantable access ports: a multivariate analysis of 385 consecutive patients. Ann Surg Oncol 15:1124–1129

Hennes R, Hofmann H (2016) Ports. Springer. ISBN 978-3-662-43640-0

Walser EM (2012) Venous access ports: indications, implantation technique, follow- up, and complications. Cardiovasc Intervent Radiol 35:751

Part V

Management of Complications in Port Procedures

Intraoperative, Postoperative, and Late Complications of Port Implantation

16

Roland Hennes

▶ **Trailer**

Mastering different strategies for complication managment associated with port systems is essential for the long-term, successful use of a central venous catheter in patients.

This chapter distinguishes between intraoperative, postoperative, and late complications of port placement. For possible intraoperative complications during port explantation, please refer to Chap. 15. Given the wide range of individual complications, we focus on the most common and clinically relevant entities.

We will not discuss infections in detail in this chapter. Infections can occur at any stage of treatment. For further information, see Chap. 7. The topic is extensively covered in the textbook "Portpflege" (Hennes and Müller 2021).

This chapter particularly focuses on technical, mechanical, and material-related complications.

R. Hennes (✉)
Klinik für Allgemein-, Viszeral- und Transplantationschirurgie, Universitätsklinikum Heidelberg, Heidelberg, Germany
e-mail: Roland.Hennes@med.uni-heidelberg.de

16.1 Intraoperative Complications

As described in Chap. 4 on indication, careful and standardized patient preparation is required to ensure an intraoperative course with as few complications as possible.

Good patient preparation minimizes complications.

Among other factors, the choice of surgical site plays a decisive role (Biffi et al. 2009). Exclusion of thrombosis, vessel obliteration, and ensuring unobstructed venous return to the heart prior to surgery are crucial for a smooth intraoperative course. In addition to the choice of surgical site, the selection of the surgical technique—specifically, whether to puncture the subclavian vein or perform a venous cutdown of the cephalic vein—is decicive for intraoperative pneumothorax risk A randomized, prospective multicenter study (Hüttner et al. 2019) comparing cephalic vein cutdown with subclavian vein puncturedemonstrated pneumothorax to be directly associated to the puncture technique. Placement of a port catheter in the cephalic vein via venous cutdown does not cause pneumothorax (Fig. 16.1).

Risks associated with comorbidities, in terms of internal medicine symptoms, must be carefully evaluated preoperatively. These will not be discussed further in this chapter.

R. Hennes (ed.), *Port Surgery*, https://doi.org/10.1007/978-3-662-70624-4_16

Management of Vascular Alterations

One of the most common challenges and resulting complications are vascular alterations, which may manifest as vessel disruption, obliteration, or extra-anatomic courses, particularly in the context of thrombosis or previous surgeries. As described in Chap. 14, we use the modified Seldinger technique as an advanced standard method to utilize small vessels as narrow as 0.5 mm for port placement. Vascular branches along the cephalic vein to the subclavian vein can also be navigated using a guidewire. This technique may be applied to all other catheter implantations sites, such as the femoral-, external- and internal jugular veins.

Simple yet clinically relevant mechanical complications include kinking of the catheter along its course.

16.1.1 Case Example 1: Sero-pneumothorax after Puncture of the Subclavian Vein

Figure 16.1 clearly shows the development of a sero-pneumothorax following puncture during central venous catheter placement. The red markings indicate the sero-pneumothorax.

16.1.2 Case Example 2: Catheter Kinking during Advancement of the Port Catheter

This situation can be resolved by simply retracting and then re-advancing the catheter; if the problem recurs, a guidewire can facilitate catheter straigtening. Deliberately advancing the kink

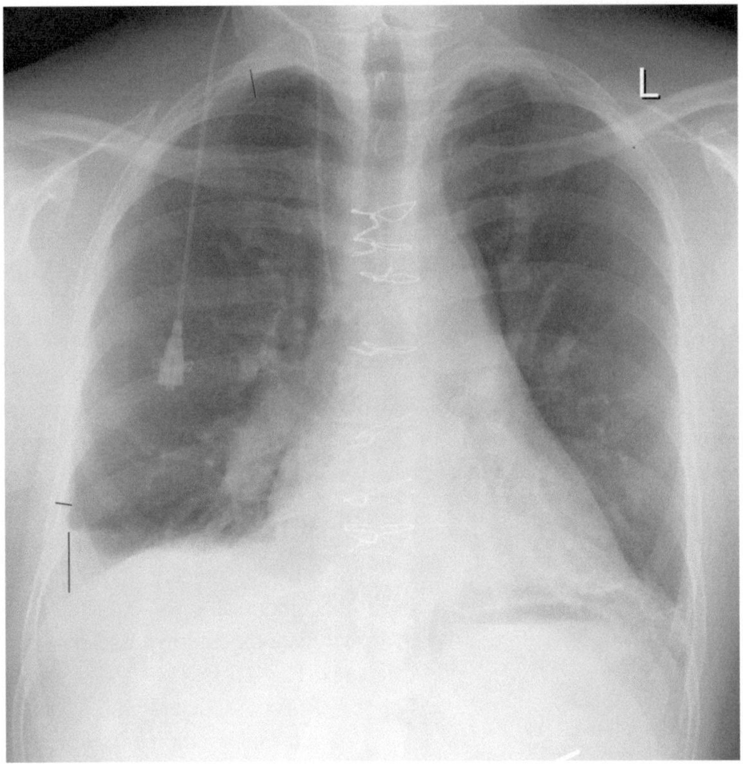

Fig. 16.1 Sero-pneumothorax after puncture. The red markings indicate the extent of the sero-pneumothorax.

into the atrium and then immediately withdrawing it can also straighten the catheter (Fig. 16.2).

16.1.3 Case Study 3: Malposition in the Azygos Vein, Internal Mammary Vein, and Pulmonary Veins

These malpositions of the port catheter are rare (approximately 1 in 2000 catheter placements), but they pose a serious problem for the patient and require urgent revision and correction (Ho et al. 2009; Talukder et al. 2017).

The most common malpositions involve the internal mammary vein (Fig. 16.3). Intraoperatively, fluoroscopy in a single imaging plane cannot precisely verify vein patency; definitive confirmation requires thoracic CT with vascular imaging. However, this is irrelevant during surgery—the critical factor is recognizing malposition. The insidious nature of this complication lies in the port catheter's unremarkable appearance on intraoperative fluoroscopy despite non-central positioning away from the atrium; blood aspiration may still be possible, but the catheter remains incorrectly placed.

In the present case, the malposition was immediately recognized because we briefly use continuous fluoroscopy to position the tip of the port catheter. If the port catheter is located in front of the atrium, i.e., centrally, the catheter

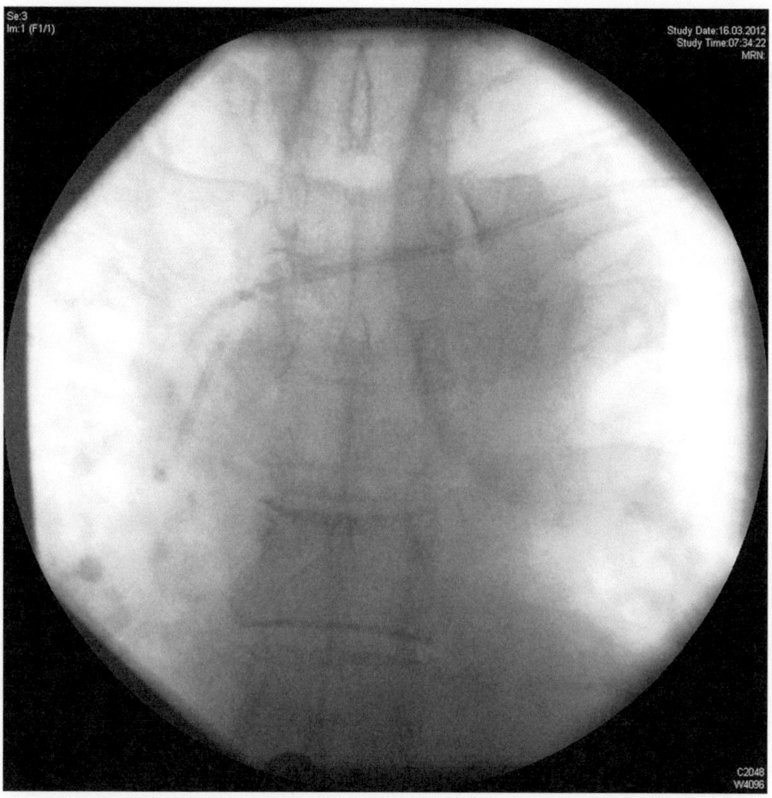

Fig. 16.2 Kinking of the catheter during advancement toward the atrium of the heart. (© R. Hennes; all rights reserved)

"swings" in rhythm with the heartbeat. This is proof of correct central placement. In this case, it did not. In our clinic, every surgeon routinely verifies correct port catheter positioning. For optimal demonstration, contrast medium is injected intraoperatively into the port catheter, clearly revealing reflux. (Fig. 16.4). Figure 16.5 shows the position of the port catheter in front of the atrium after correction. In Fig. 16.6, another malposition is demonstrated, presumably into a pulmonary vein.

> **Practical Tip** To verify the safe placement of the port catheter in front of the atrium, brief intraoperative continuous fluoroscopy should be used. This allows the rhythmic movement of the port catheter with the heartbeat to be observed.

16.1.4 Case Study 4

A typical situation during advancement of the port catheter toward the atrium is malposition in the external jugular vein (Fig. 16.7).

This malposition can be easily corrected by withdrawing the catheter back to the level of the subclavian vein. With the patient taking a deep breath, the catheter can then be advanced further. If unsuccessful, a guidewire can be introduced through the port catheter to navigate to the atrium. Alternatively, navigation can be performed using the guidewire alone, with the port catheter temporarily removed.

Port catheter looping into the external jugular vein can also occur as a late postoperative complication. Patients often report pressure sensations in the neck or head during port infusion.

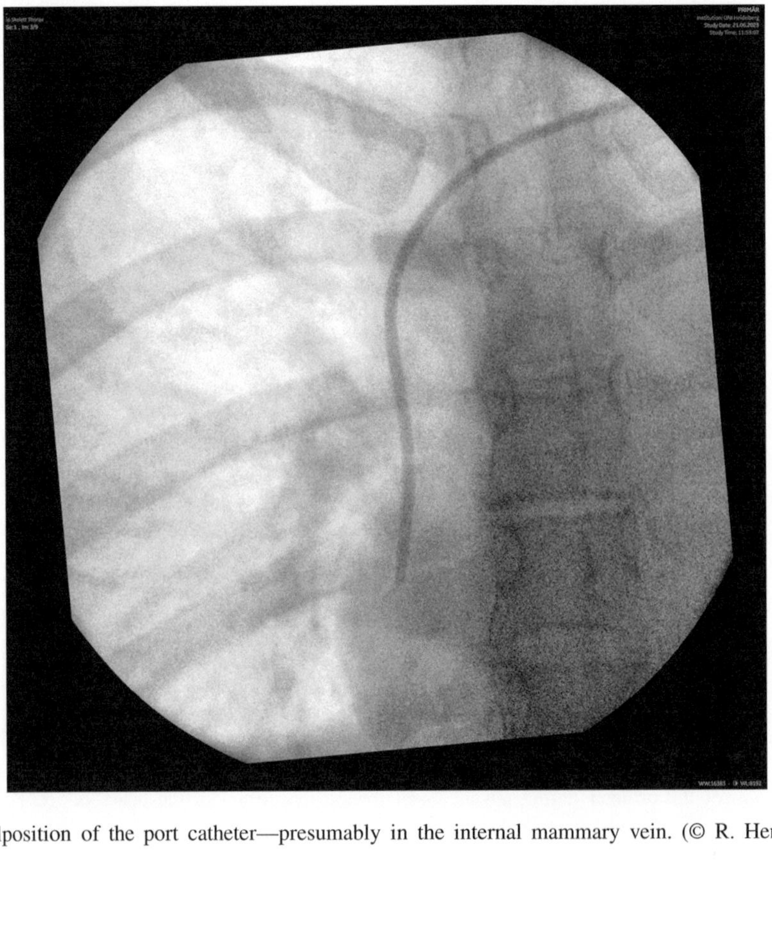

Fig. 16.3 Malposition of the port catheter—presumably in the internal mammary vein. ()

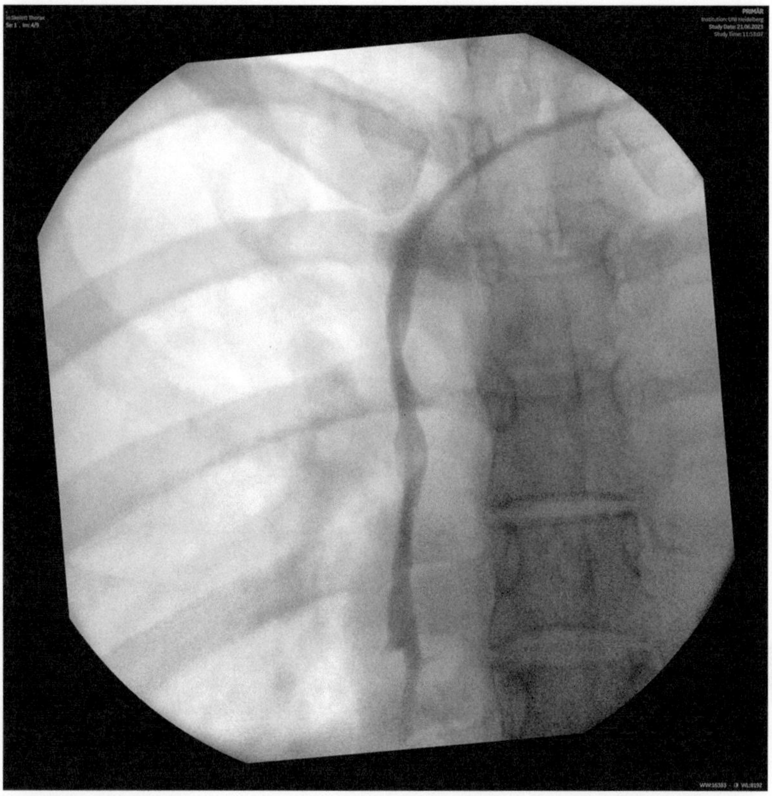

Fig. 16.4 Intraoperative administration of contrast medium to demonstrate malposition of the port catheter without outflow into the superior vena cava. (© R. Hennes; all rights reserved)

These symptoms warrant serious attention and can be confirmed via chest X-ray demonstrating jugular vein involvement.

The reasons for postoperative looping of the port catheter are often catheters that are inserted too short and do not reach the area in front of the atrium.

Coughing can cause the catheter to "swing up" and loop.

This process can be simulated intraoperatively with the patient and observed under fluoroscopy to see whether the catheter loops into the jugular vein during coughing. If this occurs, the tip of the port catheter must be advanced slightly deeper toward the atrium.

16.1.5 Case Study 5: Thrombosis Along the Subclavian and Brachiocephalic Veins

With regard to obstacles and complications that may lead to termination of implantation, venous thrombosis is of particular importance. As shown in Fig. 16.8, a thrombosis of the subclavian vein was confirmed by administration of contrast medium. This finding led to termination of the procedure. Provided no contrast medium allergy exists, intraoperative contrast administration serves as a valuable diagnostic tool to assess venous outflow and determine whether to abort the procedure or pursue port placement

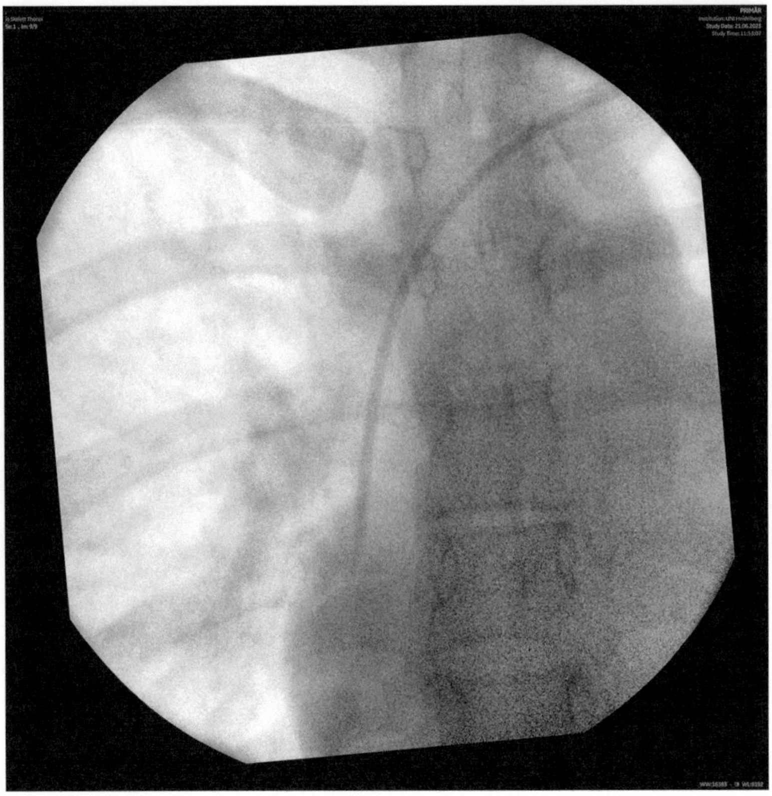

Fig. 16.5 Correct position of the port catheter in front of the atrium after repositioning and correction of the malposition. (© R. Hennes; all rights reserved)

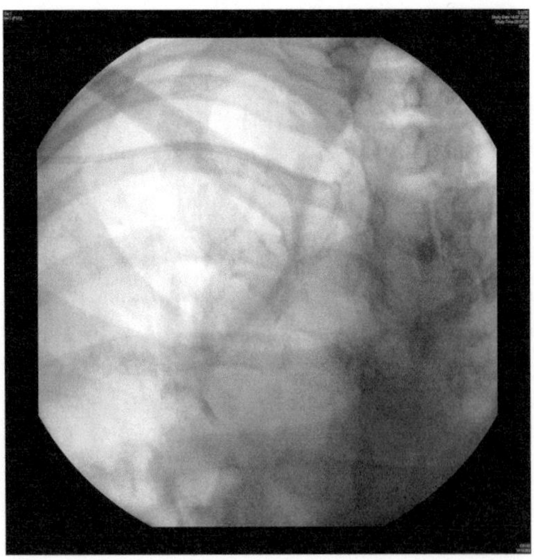

Fig. 16.6 Malposition of the port catheter, presumably branching into a pulmonary vein. (© R. Hennes; all rights reserved)

using a guidewire via the modified Seldinger technique. It bears re-emphasizing that preoperative sonographic or advanced imaging should always be performed in cases of suspected thoracic thrombosis.

16.1.6 Case Study 6: Technical Errors During Surgery

Precise knowledge and training in the use of the implantable material are essential to avoid technical errors, as illustrated in Figs. 16.9 and 16.10. In particular, soft silicone catheters are prone to kinking, whereas polyurethane catheters do not exhibit this tendency.

Due to their softness, silicone catheters can also be constricted by ligatures. This should always be checked intraoperatively.

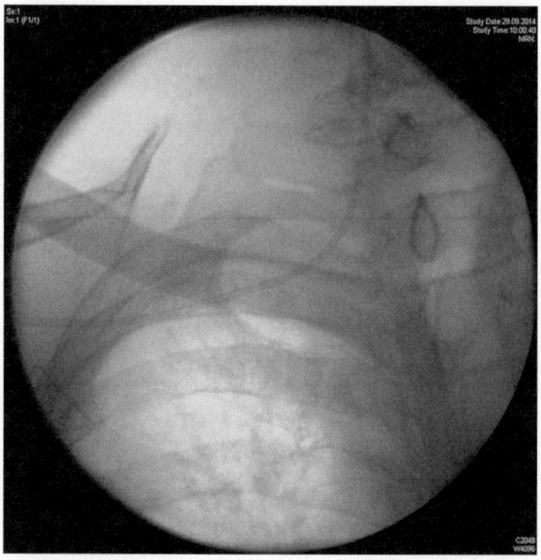

Fig. 16.7 Malposition of the port catheter due to looping of the catheter in the jugular vein. (© R. Hennes; all rights reserved)

16.2 Postoperative Complications

16.2.1 Case Study 6: Malposition of the Port Catheter in the Internal Jugular Vein

It is also possible for the catheter to flip into the internal jugular vein.

A 53-year-old female patient with breast cancer presented with port dysfunction three months after placement.

Fluoroscopy revealed that the port catheter had flipped into the internal jugular vein, resulting in kinking at the apex of the folded catheter.

Additionally, a fibrinous sheath had formed along the distal catheter segment, leading to occlusion of the catheter opening. Retrograde contrast agent extravasation could be observed

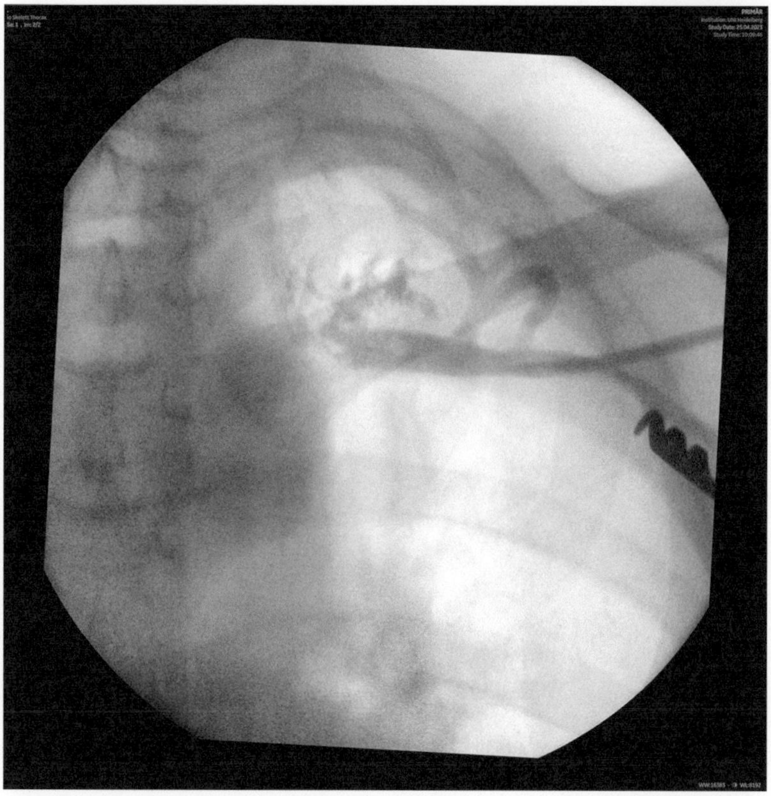

Fig. 16.8 Thrombosis along the subclavian vein with interruption of venous outflow. (© R. Hennes; all rights reserved)

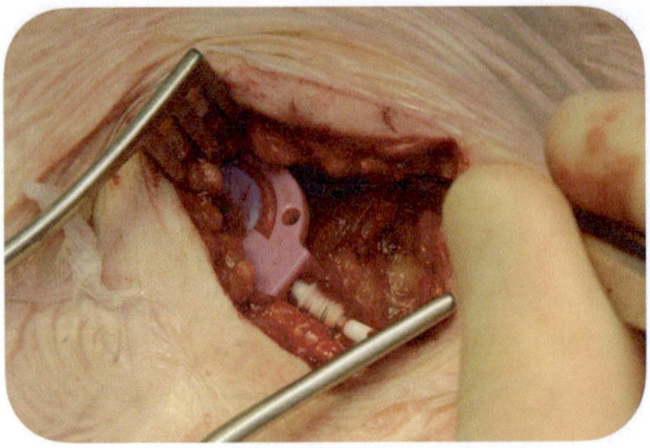

Fig. 16.9 Technical surgical error: Tilted port chamber due to lack of fixation on the fascia of the pectoralis major muscle. (© R. Hennes; all rights reserved)

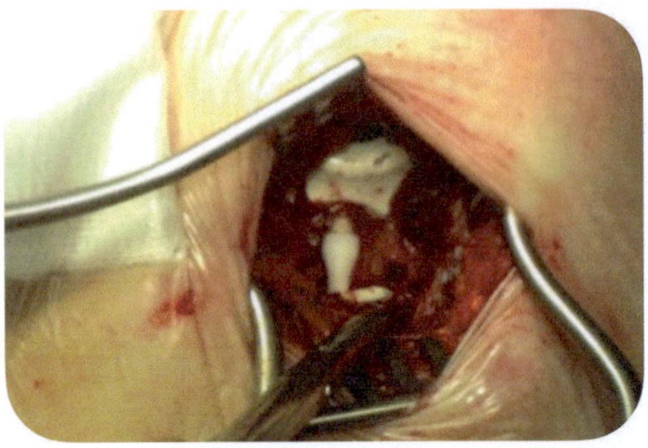

Fig. 16.10 Technical surgical error: Kinking of the port catheter behind the port coupling. (© R. Hennes; all rights reserved)

at perforations of the fibrinous sheath at the level of the distal catheter in the left brachiocephalic vein (Fig. 16.11).

16.2.2 Case Study 7: Fracture of the Port Catheter in an Arm Port

The striking example of a fractured catheter with extravasation is a recurring complication that we also frequently observe with PICC lines (Fig. 16.12). This material fatigue is clearly caused by mechanical overuse due to flexion of the arm.

16.2.3 Case Study 8: Catheter Malposition

Retraction of the port catheter with loop formation and malposition is a rare phenomenon. Patient complaints during port use—such as sensations of pressure and swelling—warrant prompt evaluation (Fig. 16.13).

16.3 Late Complications

16.3.1 Case Study 9: Incorrect Selection of Port Chamber

Incorrect selection of the port chamber size can have serious consequences for the patient. Pressure ulcers with protrusion of the port chamber through the skin regularly lead to infections that necessitate immediate revision or port explantation. Therefore barious port chamber sizes should be kept available to

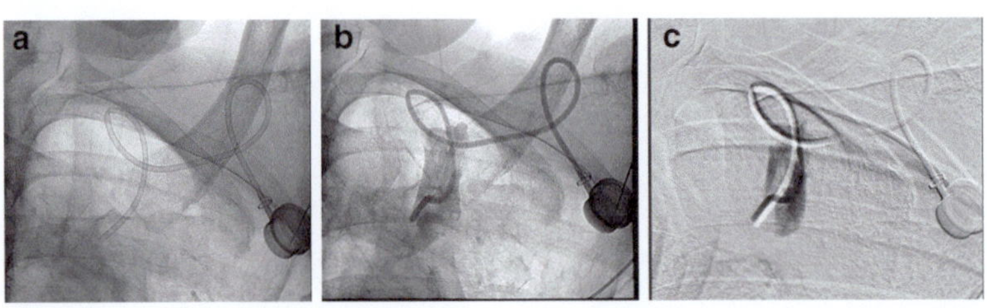

Fig. 16.11 **a–c** Port dysfunction three months after port placement: Catheter has flipped into the internal jugular vein with kinking at the apex of the folded catheter. Additionally, formation of a fibrin sheath. (© R. Hennes; all rights reserved)

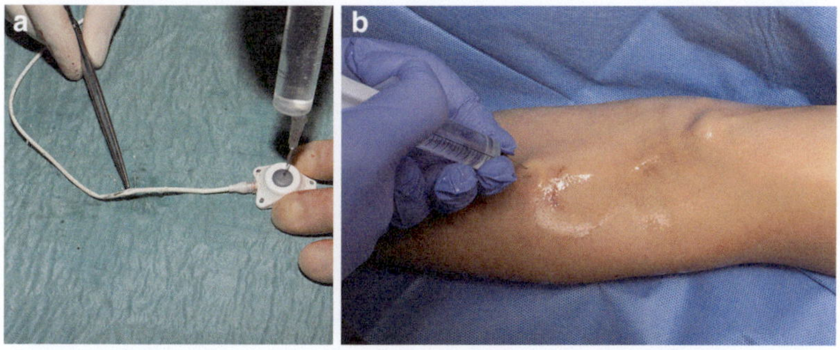

Fig. 16.12 **a,b** Fracture of the port catheter with extravasation. (© R. Hennes; all rights reserved)

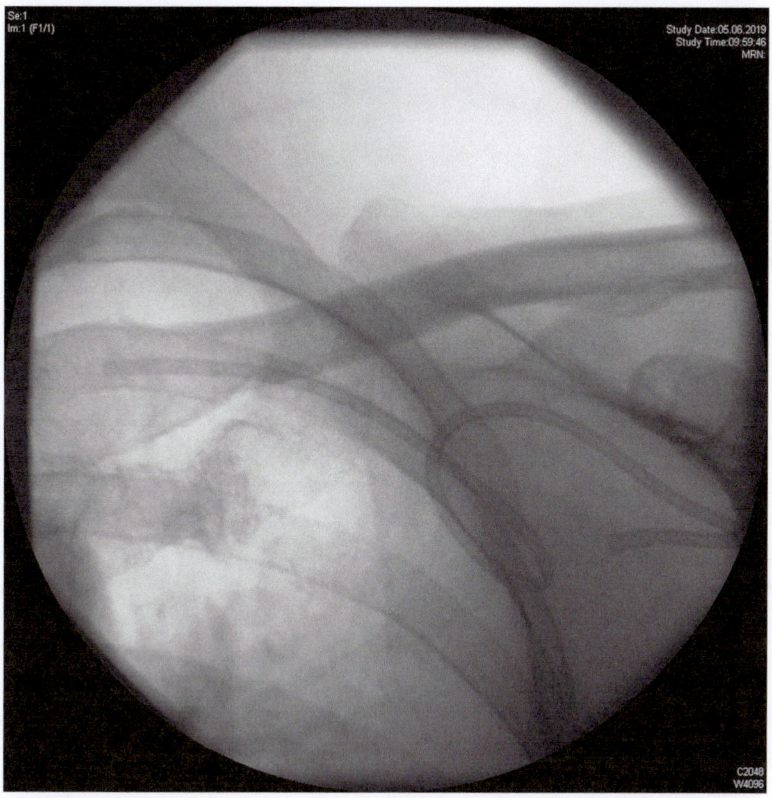

Fig. 16.13 Malposition due to "retraction" of the port catheter. (© R. Hennes; all rights reserved)

accommodate the patient's body habitus. If only one size is available, the port pocket and chamber location must be selected with care.

In very slender patients, the port chamber can also be placed deeper into the musculature of the pectoralis major to avoid f pressure ulcers caused by the port chamber. The migration of a port chamber is shown in Fig. 16.14.

16.3.2 Case Study 10: Material Fatigue

Ports remaining in situ for more than 5 years—or even over 10 years—often exhibit clear signs of material fatigue. See also Chap. 3.

Over the years, ports are exposed to a variety of stresses:

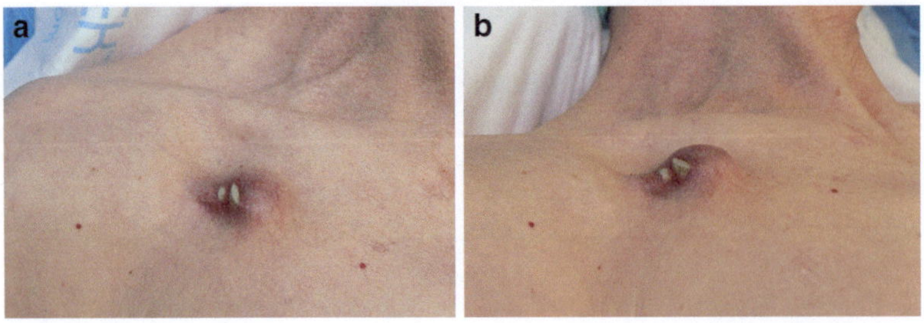

Fig. 16.14 a,b Migration of the port chamber through the skin. (© R. Hennes; all rights reserved)

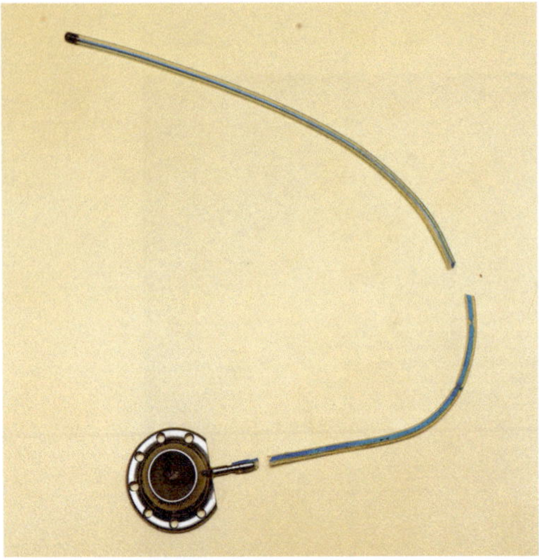

Fig. 16.15 12-year-old catheter with catheter fracture. Interventional retrieval of the catheter. (© R. Hennes; all rights reserved)

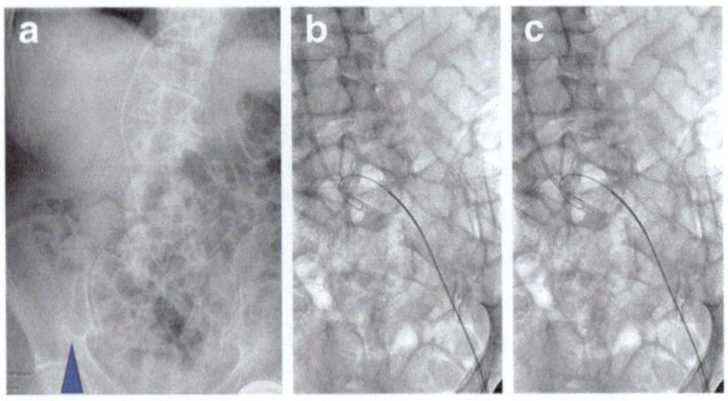

Fig. 16.16 a–c Incidental finding of a fractured catheter that could be retrieved interventionally. (© R. Hennes; all rights reserved)

including chemotherapy agents, nutritional solutions, locking solutions, and repeatedly alcohol-based solutions, all of which can directly damage the catheter material. Our recommendation is to replace or remove the port after 5 years if it is no longer needed (Fig. 16.15). Fig. 16.16a–c shows another example of material fatigue.

16.3.3 Case Study 11: Severe Intraluminal Adhesions of the Port Catheter

Chapter 15 has already addressed the problem of adhesions between the port catheter and the vascular system. Adhesions can occur especially amongst port catheters that have remained in situ for many years. It may be useful to perform a phlebography or CT scan beforehand to assess the extent of adhesions. Fig. 16.17 shows an example with particularly severe adhesions. During removal of the catheter, a small tear occurred in the brachiocephalic vein (Fig. 16.18) as a contained perforation, which could, however, be managed conservatively. The patient recovered from this complication without further symptoms or sequelae. Such a rare complication demonstrates, however, that port removals with severe adhesions can be associated with significant, potentially life-threatening complications.

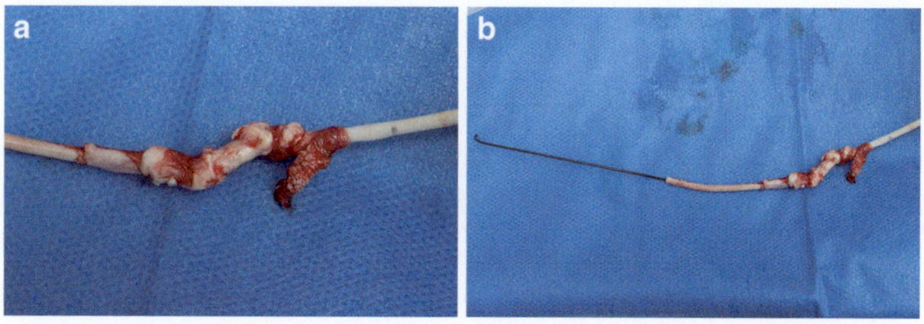

Fig. 16.17 **a,b** Severely adherent port catheter that could be retrieved using a guidewire. (© R. Hennes; all rights reserved)

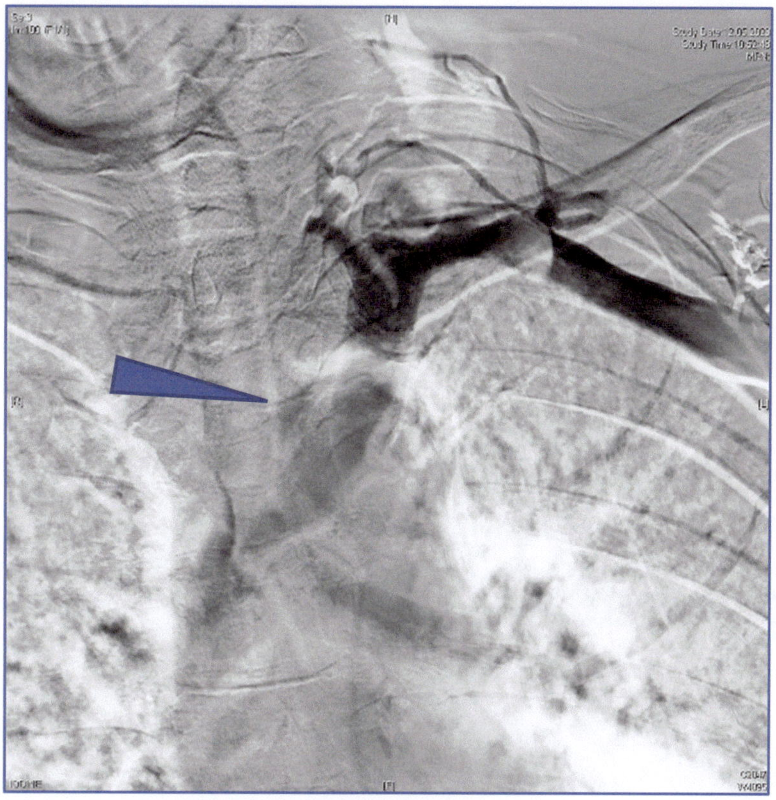

Fig. 16.18 Tear of the brachiocephalic vein with contained perforation. The blue arrow indicates the site of perforation. (© R. Hennes; all rights reserved)

References

Biffi R, Orsi F, Pozzi S et al (2009) Best choice of central venous insertion site for the prevention of catheter-related complications in adult patients who need cancer therapy: a randomized trial. Ann Oncol 20:935–940

Hennes R, Müller G (2021) Portpflege. Springe. ISBN 978-3-662-60482-3

Ho M-L, Bhalla S, Bierhals A, Gutierrez F (2009) MDCT of Partial Anomalous Pulmonary Venous Return (PAPVR) in Adults. J Thorac Imaging 24:89–95

Lyen S, Wijesuriya S, Ngan-Soo E, Mathias H, Yeong M, Hamilton M, Manghat N, Lyen et al (2017) Anomalous pulmonary venous drainage: a pictorial essay with a CT focus. Journal of Congenital Cardiology 1:7. https://doi.org/10.1186/s40949-017-0008-4

Talukder S, Srinath SR, Behera A, Ganeshan D (2017) Accidental Catheterization of Left Partial Anomalous Pulmonary Venous Connection (PAPVC): A Rare Instance of Central Venous Access Malpositioning. J Cardiovascular Thoracic Surgery. 2(3):1–3. https://doi.org/10.15226/2573-864X/2/3/00116

Part VI

Documentation and Economic Aspects

17 Economic Aspects of Port Procedures in Outpatient and Inpatient Settings

Roland Hennes

▶ Central venous catheters are playing an increasingly central role in oncology and nutritional medicine for the treatment of patients. Particularly oncologic patients benefit long-term from port systems, derive long-term benefits from port systems, which improve quality of life and maximize freedom of movement for daily activities. Although the importance of port systems is widely recognized, challenges persist in efficiently and economically representing this procedure in both outpatient and inpatient billing contexts. This chapter examines several key aspects of this issue.

According to the German Association of Epidemiological Cancer Registries, 520,000 new oncological cases were registered in Germany in 2021, with the trend continuing to rise. Data from the German Cancer Research Center in Heidelberg (DKFZ) also show increasing numbers, now well exceeding half a million new cancer cases per year in Germany. This results in the need for approximately 180,000 port implantation procedures.

R. Hennes (✉)
Klinik für Allgemein-, Viszeral- und Transplantationschirurgie, Universitätsklinikum Heidelberg, Heidelberg, Germany
e-mail: Roland.Hennes@med.uni-heidelberg.de

In addition to port catheters, related systems such as Hickman catheters and PICC lines are used. However, port catheters demonstrate the lowest infection rates and offer the highest quality of life for physical activities. In contrast, PICC lines have a manufacturer-recommended dwell time of only 3 months, while Hickman catheters—as tunneled externalized nutrition lines—preclude activities like swimming, exhibit higher infection rates, and have significantly shorter dwell times.

While demand for port implantation and central venous catheter procedures remains high, few surgeons specialize exclusively in this field. Consequently, small- and medium-sized hospitals often manage low annual case volumes, resulting in insufficient experience and expertise for complex or challenging venous conditions. Additionally, many surgeons view port implantation as a "simple" beginner's procedure—a notion that must be firmly refuted. For high-quality cancer care, central venous port catheter placement represents a demanding and critical surgical intervention that ensures successful subsequent outpatient and inpatient treatments.

To ensure efficient and economical representation of port implantation procedures, a well-conceived, consistently applied standard is required—encompassing the surgical setting, operative techniques, and postoperative care in line with best practices and evidence. (Vonlanthen R 2011).

R. Hennes (ed.), *Port Surgery*, https://doi.org/10.1007/978-3-662-70624-4_17

In the PORTAS-3 study (Hüttner et al. 2019) puncture- and venous cutdown technique were compared. Regarding complications and outcomes, the findings were clear: the evidence supports using the venous cutdown technique as the standard approach for initial port implantation, as it provides distinct advantages in reducing complication rates. In terms of cost-effectiveness, the surgeon's experience and skill play a critical role in the overall efficiency and economic impact of port procedures. In an observational study (Werba, Hennes 2023) involving 149 patients, cost-effectiveness was examined in detail, confirming an average skin-to-skin time of 10–15 min for port implantation in experienced hands. This must be considered in the context of the cost per operating minute, which averages about €100, depending on whether the procedure is performed in an outpatient setting or a central operating room. A standardized technique with an average skin-to-skin time of 15 minutes—compared to the 40 minutes typically observed in many hospitals—can have a substantial impact on the cost-effectiveness of the procedure.

Drawing on experience from more than 20,000 central venous catheter procedures—primarily port implantations—it can be stated that most patients tolerate the procedure well under local anesthesia. When required, additional analgesosedation or, in select cases, general anesthesia is administered for patients experiencing significant psychological distress. However, this remains an exception at the Port Center Heidelberg. In 2023, of 1,798 central venous catheter procedures performed at the center, only 73 patients required analgesosedation or general anesthesia for port placement. All other patients underwent the procedure under local anesthesia, having the key advantage of eliminating the need for additional anesthesia personnel.

Whenever possible, port procedures should be performed in an outpatient clinic to relieve the main operating theater. Ideally, port implantation should be performed in a dedicated outpatient operating room. Most hospitals have access to outpatient surgical areas that are spatially separated from the main operating theater. Utilizing these facilities should be strongly recommended to improve overall cost-effectiveness.

This is also confirmed at the Port Center Heidelberg: intraoperative complications, particularly infections, are rare, even among complex patients who must be operated on while aplastic or significantly immunosuppressed.

To avoid other surgical complications such as catheter malposition and lung injury, we recommend performing the procedure under intraoperative fluoroscopic guidance. When using the puncture technique, ultrasound guidance is warrented. These recommendations are particularly relevant for re-implantations and for patients with thrombosis or a history of previous port procedures, where fluoroscopic and ultrasound guidance play a crucial role in preventing complications. It should also be emphasized that exclusive reliance on ECG guidance in certain outpatient surgical settings is inherently limited. If the catheter follows an extra-anatomical course or encounters an obstruction, correct positioning of the port catheter cannot be ensured without fluoroscopic verification. This highlights the essential need for a mobile C-arm when performing ECG-guided procedures.

Billing

The procedure for placing central venous cathetersis regulated under Outpatient Surgery § 105. When port catheter placement is performed in an inpatient setting, it is billed as part of the services related to the patient's primary diagnosis. For partial inpatient admission with exclusive surgical management of the central venous system, the procedure can be billed. Therefore, careful planning of the procedure under § 105 should be carried out in outpatient practices and facilities as well as in hospital settings.

Billing for a Port Operation under § 115b

For port placement, the material costs of the procedure can be billed separately.

The following figures are guidelines for materials and equipment, as would be required for an operating room designed for the placement of central venous catheters.

Investment Requirements

1 fluoroscopy X-ray unit (C-arm)	approx. €60,000
5 instrument sets with 19 instruments each	approx. €1,500 each
1 operating table	approx. €30,000–40,000
1 surgical light	approx. €14,000
In addition, consumables such as the port, as a high-pressure port (depending on quantity and manufacturer)	approx. €80–120
1 drape kit for surgery and dressing	approx. €25.00
Puncture set	approx. €20.00
Guidewire	approx. €18–25.00
Contrast agent	approx. €2.50
Port needles	approx. €4.50
Sterilization per instrument set	approx. €12.00

Additional costs include documentation with computers and other equipment.

The introduction of a surgical kit for port procedures, especially with an appropriate case volume, has proven extremely effective at the Port Center Heidelberg. This kit includes surgical gowns, gloves, sutures, compresses, and syringes. This reduces standard time required for the procedure is significantly. Measurements at the Port Center have shown that preparing the operating table for a port procedure takes approximately 5–7 minutes. This efficiency results in a significant reduction in overall operating room time and a corresponding decrease in OR utilization minutes.

With sufficient case numbers and a good network including in and outpatient oncological clinics, the establishment of a centralized port center is economically attractive. In this context, such a center should ideally be located in major urban areas or within the catchment region of oncology clinics. Centralizing services in a dedicated port center ensures better continuity of patient care, with low complication rates, high quality of care, and consequently, optimized patient satisfaction. In this context, hygienic and legal aspects, as well as expert knowledge of the materials, are essential (Hennes and Müller 2021).

Both surgical techniques and the care of port patients should continue to evolve through the implementation of new quality standards that promote excellence in surgery and evidence-based, skilled nursing care. Advancing in this direction will enhance the overall quality of care and improve patients' quality of life, while also fulfilling economic and efficiency requirements..

References

Hennes R, Müller G (2021) Portpflege. Springer. ISBN978-3-662-60482-3

Hennes R (2023) PMCF Beobachtungstudie, in Veröffentlichung

Hüttner et al. (2019) Primary open versus closed implantation strategy for totally implantable venous access ports. Ann Surg

Vonlanthen R, Slankamenac K, Breitenstein S et al (2011) The impact of complications on costs of major surgical procedures: a cost analysis of 1200 patients. Ann Surg 254:907–913

MIX
Papier aus verantwortungsvollen Quellen
Paper from responsible sources
FSC® C105338

If you have any concerns about our products,
you can contact us on
ProductSafety@springernature.com

In case Publisher is established outside the EU,
the EU authorized representative is:
Springer Nature Customer Service Center GmbH
Europaplatz 3, 69115 Heidelberg, Germany

Printed by Libri Plureos GmbH
in Hamburg, Germany